The Glutathione Book

Creating The Holy Grail of Supplements –
Our Challenge To Build The Market's First
Functional Glutathione Product

Dan Purser MD

By Dan Purser MD

Physician/Practitioner

Bestselling Author

Educator

Supplement Designer/Developer

PhysicianDesigned.com

DanPurserMd.com

PhysicianDesigned.com

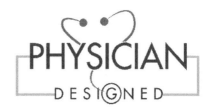

Preface

This product, a working oral glutathione, had to be created. The world of medicine, and the health of a lot of people, required it.

We did it. My formulating partner (the amazing Steve Pitcher) and I, created the mother of all anti-oxidants. It took us a year of late nights, many hundreds of hours of discussions, and lots of sweat. We then confirmed it with our validation testing (see the chapter on articles – our white paper from our validation work is in there).

Who could benefit from this?

Most people actually, because they have lost the ability to reduce glutathione either due to age or toxin trauma. All the genetic errors out there need it including all the kids with autism. Any severe burn, chronic renal failure patients, viral infection sufferers, anyone with fibromyalgia, or those with heavy metal problems – reduced glutathione is critical to the functionality of the metallothionien.

Steve and I made this for you – all of you.

This is the most amazing product and this is the road and the map we took to travel that path to success.

Thanks for reading.

– Dan Purser, MD

Disclaimers

Income Disclaimer

This document contains health and business strategies, marketing methods, and other business advice that, regardless of my own results and experience, may not produce the same results (or any results) for you. I make absolutely no guarantee, expressed or implied, that by following the advice below you will make any money or improve current profits, as there are several factors and variables that come into play regarding any given business.

Primarily, results will depend on the nature of the product or business model, the conditions of the marketplace, the experience of the individual, and situations and elements that are beyond your control.

As with any business endeavour, you assume all risks related to investment of money based on your own discretion and at your own potential expense.

Liability Disclaimer

By reading this document, you assume all risks associated with using the advice given below, with a full understanding that you, solely, are responsible for anything that may occur as a result of putting this information into action in any way, and regardless of your interpretation of the advice.

You further agree that our company cannot be held responsible in any way for the success or failure of your business as a result of the information presented below. It is your responsibility to conduct your own due diligence regarding the safe and successful operation of your business if you intend to apply any of our information in any way to your business operations.

Terms of Use

You are given a non-transferable, "personal use" license to this product. You cannot distribute it or share it with other individuals.

Also, there are no resale rights or private label rights granted when purchasing this document. In other words, it's for your own personal use only.

Dedication

I dedicate this to Coleman and Merry Caroline
Purser, two of my most amazing children –
I created this for you and your future.

Thank you for always being you.

Table of Contents

Chapter 1

My Rules For A Functional Glutathione Supplement, Why, & Why Now?

The "Why" First

We have a problem. Well, actually you have a problem.

There's a ton of useless glutathione products in the marketplace – the ones we looked at or tested were a joke – they didn't work. Period.

We haven't been the only ones who noticed. It's a problem.

We call this problem "background noise" because the non-working ones steal market share, and the market noise they create block out the real one (ours) that works. You can also call it a waste of money.

Or some might actually call this a tragedy – in today's toxic environment and world, people need a functional glutathione that works – really works. As in, raises blood levels. As in, you can feel the glutathione and how it clears your head out and makes you feel amazing!

So Why Now?

Because people are so much smarter then ever before – we have so much more knowledge.

Also, a lot of us are learning our genetic issues (get your 23andme® and and Nutrahacker® to see what I mean). Or they get intracellular levels in Spectracell® Comprehensive Micronutrient results that indicate they have a low intracellular level of glutathione.

How do I know this?
Because my book on genetic errors (called **The 85% Solution: MTHFR is Overpowering Our Medical System – Chances Are You Have It Too...**), problems like MTHFR, COMT, and GSTP1 was a huge massive bestseller on Amazon® – Amazon® Top50® and Amazon® Top 100® and the top book in the Healthcare and Medical categories on Amazon® in the summer of 2016, I ended up talking to a LOT of patients and people in regard to these concepts. And the majority of these people had genetic errors that suggestes they'd benefit from a functional glutathione.

Then they'd ask their doctor what they should take – the doctor says NAC or cysteine but their intracellular level would never change. Then they would buy one of the background noise products off the internet or at a local healthfood store – it does not work – and still, their levels are the same. They do not feel any better. They feel ripped off. Cheated.

I've also spoken about health issues all over the planet the last few years (it helps to develop popular products and to write #1 books), and I've heard it over and over from practitioners (MDs, nurse practitioners, naturopaths, chiropractors) in Japan, Malaysia, Australia, Europe, and in all the states of the USA, that there is no workable or functional glutathione – when was I going to figure this out?

The other interesting secret, that most people miss, is that a real functional glutathione is incredibly valuable. Think about it – it could be used for macular degeneration (the #1 cause of blindness in the world), for HIV or AIDS patients who desparately need it, burn patients who cannot make it, kidney failure patients who could possibly be saved from dialysis, and more. Much, MUCH more.

A functional glutathione is THAT valuable – it's worth billions and billions of dollars.

The challenge had been laid down.

My partner, Steve Pitcher, and I had the ultimate product to develop. It was indeed the holy grail of supplements.

We always develop real products that work.

This HAD to be one of those.

We then test and validate those products and post or publish the results. That's called validation or verification. We also protect or products with patents – expensive, but necessary. Why?

There's a ton of useless glutathione products out there, and our competition does not know how to make one that works.

We felt like we could because of our past glutathione research.

So we would patent it (if we could). But I'm repeating myself.

We've worked more with glutathione than any humans on the planet – even been involved in an incredible patented nanoized version (technically a drug, so forget it as a supplement). We also know that Bastyr University (Washington) performed a landmark study on oral glutathione – the ones they tested did not work. None of them. Why? There's a ton of useless glutathione products out there – but, hey, I'm repeating myself.

Rules, Rules, Rules…

Through years of at looking at products that do not work, we have slowly developed rules for a mythical glutathione that could and would work.

What are our twelve rules for designing a workable affordable glutathione?

A functional glutathione:

1. Must be **oral**.
2. Must be **affordable**.
3. Must be easily **accessible.**
4. Must be **reduced**.
5. The reduced GSH must be **stable** (i.e. protected from oxidation – triiiiicky, and where almost all our competitors fall down).
6. Must have a tolerable **taste** (ours does – we used lemon and mint essential oils)
7. Must be all **natural** – ours is that (we use a super high quality all natural GSH out of Japan).
8. Must have an adequate **dose** – ours has an INCREDIBLE 1100mg of Glutathione per serving (550mg as liposome embedded GSH). For

Amazon competition numbers, we had to be the best, so we went beyond everyone else and maxed out the liposome – they cannot hold more than this.

9. Must be in an **airtight bottle** (or it will oxidize with oxygen in the air and be worthless).

10. Must be **validated** (38% rise in GSH levels day one. 50+% improvement in GSH/GSSG ratios after a month. Are you kidding us? The data is posted on our website. Is theirs?).

11. **FDA drug status capable** – good enough to seek drug status with a modified topical version. Is theirs good enough (no, theirs don't even work – see Bastyr study) to try to apply for various drug applications? (Ours is, so we're gearing up to spend upwards of a paltry $30 million in the next year or two.)

Let's break these down one by one.

#1 Must be **oral.**

Oral supplemenets are usually not a problem – not a problem in the sense that the FDA does not consider them to be a problem. By definition they are usually a supplement (unless the product in question has been registered as a medicine some time in the past).

Topical applications are usually considered a drug by the FDA (unless it's a cosmetic – that has very few regulation ties to it). But hoping for absorption and functionality through the skin makes a supplement, what ever it is, defined by the FDA, as a drug.

Now glutathione itself, is considered to be a supplement – it is considered to be GRAS/E by the FDA (Generally Regarded As Safe/Effective) though no monograph had been written on it (a bizarre situation). We discovered this when we first talked to the FDA – hopefully this has been remedied (by lW a monograph is required on all supplemenets).

Again, a cosmetic is fairly strictly defined: "The Federal Food, Drug, and Cosmetic Act (FD&C Act) defines cosmetics by their intended use, as *"articles intended to be rubbed, poured, sprinkled, or sprayed on, introduced into, or otherwise applied to the human body...for cleansing, beautifying, promoting attractiveness, or altering the appearance"* [FD&C Act, sec. 201(i)]. Among the products included in this definition are skin moisturizers, perfumes, lipsticks, fingernail polishes, eye and facial makeup preparations, cleansing shampoos, permanent waves, hair colors, and deodorants, as well as any substance intended for use as a component of a cosmetic product."[1]

Topical drugs have a broad set of definitons – go to: http://www.fda.gov/drugs/developmentapprovalproces s/howdrugsaredevelopedandapproved/approvalapplica tions/over-the-counterdrugs/default.htm for more information on this subject. We dealt with an excellent patented topical glutathione (complexed form), but in the end we had to abandon it because as a supplement it just was too awkward and legally problematic with which to deal.

"Legal vitamins" must be listed by the FDA as a supplement, and then need to be orally taken and absorbed to be allowed into the marketplace.

We had to find an oral glutathione – there were thirty to fifty or more on the market.

#2 Must be **affordable.**

For a supplement to work it must be reasonably and competitively priced – this means it needs to be reasonable to manufacture.

What do I mean by this?

Let's look at this in the extreme.

No one will buy a $1,000 a bottle product. Or very, very few will. Even if it is the holy grail product. Even if it does all the things we've actually determined a real functional glutathione will do – things no one else knows, or has written about because they've never had a workable glutathione before (more on these mysterious benefits later). You could sell it for $1 but then you could not manufacture it for very long – you'd be out of business before you knew it.

So most of the reasonable (remember that they still don't work) glutathiones on the market are being sold at just under $50 – so that seemed like a reasonable price. We just had to be able to make our product at a multiple of less than that so we could get it to market.

#3 Must be easily **accessible.**

Accessibility must be a requirement, because if no one could get their hands on a product, it would never sell – again it would not benefit the world and you would not be in business very long, if at all.

For example injectable or IV glutathione are both accessible, however they are not *easily* accessible. Mainly because you'd need to visit a doctor who'd be willing to order it in a prescription (good luck), and second you'd have to find a pharmacy in which to fill the prescription. Both are significant hurdles.

Buying online or at your local health food store is easy and makes it very accessible.

We had to design something that could sell online or retail somewhere.

Being available in retail or online would be a very competitive situation since there are probably fifty or more glutathione products out there and the background noise (the main trouble with developing a real product that actually works) is a real problem with glutathione.

So we felt we could make whatever we developed accessible, we just didn't know how we could make it stand out above the crowd of non-functioanl glutathiones.

Now you know why I wrote this book.

#4 Must be **reduced.**

Reduced glutathione is called GSH (I have never been able to determine for what exactly this acronym stands though many have said it's a chemical term) – people who need glutathione supplementation usually need it because they cannot reduce used or oxidized glutathione back to GSH – i.e. see Autism Spectrum Disorder). GSH is ready to accept (starving for it actually) an oxidant, a heavy metal, a toxin, a virus, or something foreign floating around inside the body.

GSSG (chemical acronym for oxidized glutathione) is not what you want but that's mostly what you get. GSSG is not useful – it is like a bear trap that's been sprung – it's full, no room at the inn. You cannot get anything else into it because it already is loaded up. The problem is all the products out there we tested and looked at were GSSG and not GSH – they may have started as GSH but the second they were exposed to oxygen (i.e. air) they became oxidized (they aggressively bind to oxygen that's why it's call "oxidizing"), and as I've said the problem is most people cannot reduce the oxidized GSSG back to GSH (see chapters 9 and 14).

This product must be GSH. It must be reduced. And it must be protected (i.e. stable).

#5 The reduced GSH must be **stable.**

Stable, in this context means it must be protected from oxidation – triiiiicky and where almost all our competitors fall down – we partnered with a very advanced company who deals in supplements to help us do this, using their technology – but it's our idea, and our patent too.

There are a number of wayst to protect GSH from oxidation, but we used a tried and true method – we embedded the GSH within a liposome.

Liposomes are not a new technology and not a new carrier for glutathione. And people can readily absorn GSH from a liposome (topically or orally).

But there are two problems with using liposomes. First, the manufacturing process itself must be carefully planned and held to, so that as the liposome is built around the GSH molecule everything stays oxygen free (trying doing that in an aqueous environment) – so we developed a pateneted process for the manufacturing. Second, the handling and bottling must be done correctly – an airtight bottle (we saw none, with this feature, in all the market ones we looked at), and the bottling process itself must be done under airless conditions.

That is how you maintain GSH in reduced state; from creation to packaging to application by the end user. It's the only way this works.

#6 Must have a tolerable **taste.**

Wow, this one is critical and very doable as long as you have an encaged, reduced, and stable GSH molecule. The glutathione products we bought on Amazon® almost all tasted horrible, especially after the bottles had been opened, used and then sat in the refrigerator a few days. It's because oxidized glutathione (GSSG) tastes horrible and smells worse, and either their product was not reduced or the bottling and pump were wrong (neither were airless, so air could get in) – but as I've said, all the ones we looked at were GSSG anyway when we opened the bottle – they had not used the correct manufacturing process in order to keep it reduced.

The flavoring, due to the advancing requirements of the end users out there (you) must be all natural, too. Again, we rarely saw that in action. Since my team had so much experience in this area, we used lemon and mint essential oils.

The other benefit of lemon essential oil is it contains d-limonene which has been shown to naturally increase GSH and GPX (glutathione peroxidase) levels. Cool!

#7 Must be all **natural.**

Like I've said previously, the marketplace has been changing, and now end users demand all natural products. Our GSH is all natural – we use a super high quality all natural GSH out of Japan called Setria®, but that's nothing super special – there are probably twenty other products out there that use the same.

Also, as I've explained in the previous section, we use an all natural (gas chromatography verified) essential oil combo for our flavoring.

Plus, our liposomes are lecithin based, so they are natural also.

#8 Must have an adequate **dose.**

Ours has an INCREDIBLE 550 mg of Glutathione per serving (550mg as liposome embedded GSH). We did this for Amazon® competition, the numbers said we had to be the best (highest) so we went above and beyond everyone else and maxed out the liposome (*a true liposomal glutathione cannot hold more than this*).

#9 Must be in an **airtight bottle**

If you don't use an impermeable bottle, the GSH will oxidize with oxygen in the air and be worthless.

The problem is airtight bottles are not cheap – they are EXPENSIVE as in $$$$$. They must be made of special oxygen proof plastic or glass (too heavy and not safe), so the oxygen cannot get in to ruin the GSH. It's part of maintaining the stability of the reduced GSH in the liposome. The next problem is, due to the expense, most developers and/or manufacturers would never think of using one. We noticed no one, who claimed they had liposomal or reduced glutathione (GSH), used an actual airtight bottle. We do. It's required for a premium product that really works.

#10 Must be **validated**.

What does this mean? It means your product (OUR product in this case) has validating tests which support it benefits. WE have done multiple studies on ours, mimicking the Basyr study, and we can get an average of a 38% rise in GSH levels throughout day one (Bastyr got ZERO with product they tried and that was after 2 grams were taken orally). 50+% improvement in GSH/GSSG ratios after a month. (Are you kidding us? The data is posted on our website. Is theirs?). I also put a copy of our original study in the study/article chapter of this book. We have no fear in publishing it because it has been readily duplicated.

#11 **FDA drug status capable**.

It is good enough to seek drug status with a modified topical version. Is theirs good enough (no, theirs don't even work – see Bastyr study[2]) to try to apply for various drug applications? (Ours is, so we're gearing up to spend upwards of a paltry $30 million in the next year or two for approval as a drug. too.)

Chapter 2

Glutathione Deficiency – Why You? Why Now?

Who cares about a glutathione product? Or I guess should ask why should you care or why do you feel like you need some glutathione supplementation?

Has some physician told you? Or have you figured this out on your own?

There are several reasons why someone might need glutathione or have a deficiency of glutathione (GSH). Here they are:

1. Genetic error prevents formation of adequate amounts of glutathione (remember that we're strictly talking about GSH here).
2. Genetic errors prevent you from being able to reduce used glutathione (GSSG) back to GSH (probably the MOST COMMON reason).
3. Vitamin or nutritional deficiencies prevent adequate creation or reduction of GSH.
4. Oxidant or free radical insult overwhelms your system and overuses all your GSH, and will continue the daily overuse until the insult is withdrawn or stopped.

5. Major trauma, such as a serious burn uses up all your GSH and keeps using it.
6. You have renal failure and it uses up your GSH.
7. You have a serious viral illness such as: Hepatitis C, Hepatitis B, Epstein Barr, HIV/AIDS, Shingles, or Herpes (Type 1 or 2) that shuts off your GSH production.
8. You have excessive exposure to a heavy metal or too much of a physiologic metal (such as copper or iron) and it drops your GSH level to near zero.
9. You've had cancer and received chemotherapy and now suffer from chemo brain.
10. Type II Diabetes is associated with reduced glutathione levels – but is it a cause or an effect?

Now let's look at these in more detail.

1. Genetic errors prevents formation of adequate amounts of glutathione (remember that we're usually talking about GSH here but in this case we are talking about glutathione in general). Mainly the errors (such as GPX1 or GSTP1) prevent re-reduction of the oxidized glutathione (GSSG) to reduced glutathione (GSH or the active form of glutathione that we need to survive).

2. Genetic errors prevent you from being able to reduce used glutathione (GSSG) back to GSH (probably the MOST COMMON reason). GPX1, GSTP1, NAD2, SOD2 and others are just the tip of the iceberg.

3. Vitamin or nutritional deficiencies prevent adequate creation or reduction of GSH.

   N-Acetyl-Cysteine (or NAC), L-Glycine, or L-Glutamine deficienices are the common intracellular deficiencies I often see, which in turn cause glutathione deficiencies.

   Glutathione is a tripeptide made up of the three amino acids[3] (I mentioned above) which need to be in our diet or be made by our bodies. In my experience, NAC and Glutamine are probably the two most commonly depleted that lead to a glutathioine deficiency.

   "An **essential amino acid**, or **indispensable amino acid**, is an amino acid that cannot be synthesized *de novo* (from scratch) by the organism, and thus must be supplied in its diet. The nine amino acids humans cannot synthesize
   are phenylalanine, valine, threonine, tryptopha

n, methionine, leucine, isoleucine, lysine, and histidine (i.e., F V T W M L I K H).[1,2]

Six other amino acids are considered **conditionally essential** in the human diet, meaning their synthesis can be limited under special pathophysiological conditions, such as prematurity in the infant or individuals in severe catabolic distress.[2] These six
are arginine, cysteine, glycine, glutamine, proline, and tyrosine (i.e. R C G Q P Y)."[3]

We've known since 1953[4] or earlier (1924?) that lack of cysteine would cause a deficiency of glutathione. Most humans internally create adequate cysteine, but some people canot due to genetic errors or diseases. Thus their glutathione levels drop or are never adequate (such as children with autism[5]).

Glutamine is another amino acid critical to the manufacture of GSH, but it's "considered" a "conditionally essential" (see above) amino acid (although technically, it is not) meaning we often cannot create it and must take it in nutritionally in order to facilitate the manufacture of glutathione.

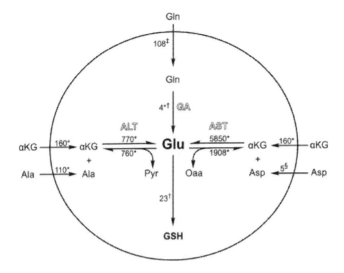

Diagram – shows the formation of glutathione then subsequent reduction to the GSH (reduced form of glutathione).

Glycine is the last critical amino acid in the formation of glutathione and it too is considered "conditionally essential" (meaning we cannot manufacture it internally under pathologic condtions such as genetic errors). It usually must be part of your diet.

B

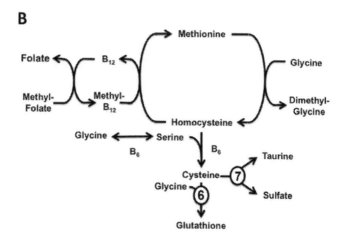

Diagram shows the formation of glutathione and how folate, methylated B12, and homocystein all eventually help in that formation.

4. Oxidant or free radical insult overwhelms your system and overuses all your GSH, and will continue the daily overuse until the insult is withdrawn or stopped.

This oxidant overload causes a significant glutathione deficiency and goes without saying, but technically we've known since the 1960s.

5. You have major trauma such as a serious burn which immediately uses up all your GSH and keeps using it.

   Burns (thermal) are the fourth most common cause of trauma worldwide[6]. Glutathione has been shown to be massively decreased in burn patients. And has also been shown to assist in burn healing (mesotherapeutic injections[7] – ouch – but they had no oral or topical version that worked – right?).

   In our reconstructive surgery office we've gotten amazing results from treating laser burns or even severely sunburned patients with our liposomal glutathione used in trials. Also the scars were dramatically decreased, to almost zero. The effect was almost immediate too, which very much surprised us.

6. You have a serious viral illness such Hepatitis C[8], Hepatitis B, Epstein Barr, HIV/AIDS, Shingles, or Herpes (Type 1 or 2) that shuts off your GSH production.

   All the above viruses (and maybe others), especially HIV, when infecting the person almost immediately turn off the production of reduced glutathione (GSH)[9]. This is because

GSH is incredibly anti-viral and we think CD4 and CD8 T-Killer white bood cells use it to attack the viruses in question.

Studies have also shown that if someone has full blown AIDS and their GSH levels reach or approach zero they usually die.

So functional glutathione is very anti-viral.

7. You have excessive exposure to a heavy metal or too much of a physiologic metal (such as copper or iron) and it drops your GSH level to near zero.

Physiologic metals (copper, chromium, etc.) and pathologic or xenobiotic metals (lead, mercury, cadmium, etc.) are removed or moved around the body by a set of enzymes known as metallothioneins. Metallothioneins in turn require functional GSH, which makes up a third of the metallothioein, to work and be effective[10].

This is why people on the AS (Autism Spectrum), suffer from heavy metal toxicity – most cannot properly reduce glutathione back to GSH (the lack glutathione peroxidase or GPx in proper amounts)[11].

8. You've had cancer and received chemotherapy and now suffer from chemo brain.

   Chemo brain occurs because of chemotoxins still residing in the brain due to lack of GSH or functional metallothioneins to remove them (see #8). We believe that using a functional absorbable GSH should alleviate this (although no data exits as of yet, though we are working on that).

9. Type II Diabetes is associated with reduced glutathione levels[12] – but is it a cause or an effect?

   Functional GSH seems to dramatically reduce Hemglobin A1C, though we're not sure why this occurs so rapidly. The GSH also seems to be associated with better renal function in diabetic patients too. More studies need to be obtained to find out why and how much.

Chapter 3

Why Glutathione Supplements Usually Don't Work

We don't know if this holds true for all glutathione supplements, we just haven't found one that is effective and really works in the competition marketplace out there. As you can tell, this is what drove us to design one that works and then to get a patent on the product.

Here are the reasons we discovered or determined:

- The product was not originally reduced (so not GSH), it's just GSSG (oxidized glutathione) – this is a manufacturing design flaw, and is the most common defect we found. The formulator/designer or manufacturer probably (clearly?) did not understand that it should be reduced and just threw the raw oxidized glutathione into a capsule or liposome and sold it. This will not affect proper blood levels at all (see the Bastyr study[13]).

- The product was originally reduced (GSH, could have even been excellent Setria® like we use) but they did not maintain the anaerobic (oxygen free) environment throughout the manufacturing process, so in the end the product is still oxidized glutathione (GSSG), and still worthless.

- The Product may have started as GSH, gone through all the right processes (but we doubt this, as ours was the first patent to claim this), but because of poor bottling, bottle design, or the wrong plastic, is no longer reduced, but oxidized from the air. Note that the wrong plastics will be readily permeable to air (oxygen) and so would ruin the GSH (if it ever was GSH). We even found a product bottled in glass (correct – they win the prize) but we did not feel it was reduced glutathione (GSH) so we are not sure why they used the glass (to look different for marketing purposes maybe?).

- The product had the wrong carrier or no carrier was utilized, thus being unable to protect the GSH after it comes out of the bottle. We used the lecithin based liposome for this version, but there are other carriers that could be used and so they are covered in our patent.

Chapter 4

Glutathione Benefits – Known

Having an adequate level of glutathione is critical to good health. It does so many things well that I will just list the ones I know off the top of my head, keeping in mind that my team has been involved with so many research projects (with just about the only functional glutathione on the planet) that it's hard to keep track.

Some of these benefits will have never before been discussed or tied to glutathione, so maybe some might find this list a bit controversial – sorry, but these are what we've observed and documented. And again, I must apologize as some of these seem a little miraculous but they are what they are.

This list also is applicable mostly when glutathione levels (and GSH/GSSG ratios) have reached optimal levels. This is a goal and process that can take weeks or months using a true functional reduced glutathione, or utilizing the same topically or transdermally (which technically makes it a drug requiring FDA approval of course).

So here it is – why people should or would want to take adequate oral or topical amounts of true functional reduced glutathione (GSH):

- Prevents cholesterol from being oxidized to plaque.

- Normalizes kidney function for most people.

- Normalizes liver function for most people.

- Prevents or reverses wet macular degeneration.

- Improves or clears up neuropathy.

- Improves diabetes and insulin receptor function.

- Stops shingles post-herpetic neuralgia from occurring.

- Stops shingles outbreak, dries up lesions.

- Reverses Hepatitis C or B liver function test elevation and reduces viral load.

- Improves EBV (Epstien Barr Virus) symptoms and helps reduce viral load.

- Stops and helps resolve herpes (Types 1& 2) outbreaks.

- Improves depression in some patients.

- Improves or resolves brain fog in most patients.

- Lightens acne scarring and inflammation.

- Helps skin wounds heal and minimizes scarring.

- Can dramatically help minor to severe burns to heal and minimize scarring.

- Reduces HIV viral load.

Chapter 5

Oral Glutathione – Why? FDA Rules Discussed

Glutathione is considered to be GRAS/E, or a legal supplement, by the FDA. GRAS/E means a supplement or product is Generally Regarded As Safe and Effective. This means it is safe and can be given to anyone. Talking to the FDA in 2014 they were surprised they did not have a monograph (rare) on glutathione (hopefully they've written this since).

For five years we were involved in research surrounding an incredible nano based or complexed product involving reduced glutathione (GSH) but it was topical. The trouble was, if we wanted to use it or sell it as a supplement, we could not, since technically the FDA considers topically absorbed supplements to be a drug unless they're deemd a cosmetic which this, as a supplement, would not be).

For a supplement to not be a drug it needs to be able to be absorbed orally – so we've designed ours accordingly.

Chapter 6

Why Reduced Glutathione?
Glutathione GSH Explained

Many humans eventually cannot make enough GSH, or some are born with this problem (genetics). The main enzyme that reduces GSSG to GSH is Glutathione Peroxidase Enzyme-1 (GPx-1, and there are three more of these peroxidase enzymes, but they tend to be minimal players). Anything that reduces your level of GPx-1 is a problem and in turn reduces GSH production.

Selenium Deficiency

Selenium deficiency may be the most common cause of GPx-1 deficiency (and thus a GSH deficiency). In human populations, selenium deficiency, due to lack of selenium in the soil, has been found to cause a heart disorder known as Keshan disease[14,15,16,17], a cardiomyopathy, and Kashin-Beck[18,19] disease[287, 393], an osteoarthropathy, in part due to reductions in GPx-1 expression.

The main sign of Keshan disease is unexplained myocardial necrosis causing a cardiomyopathy, leading to weakening of the heart. Selenium deficiency also contributes to Kashin-Beck disease, a disease that tends to result in atrophy, degeneration, and necrosis of cartilage tissue in the joints. It's important to note that many patients in our office, with a measured intraceullular glutathione deficiency (GSH), also suffer from a mild to moderate joint inflammation which they think is caused by some unexplained form of arthritis – oddly this is resolved with the taking of a functional glutathione.

Clearly a GPx-1 deficiency enhances endothelial cell activation and inflammation, especially in joints and the vascular system.

Genetic Errors Causing a GPX1 Enzyme Deficiency

Glutathione peroxidase-1 (GPx-1) is a crucial antioxidant enzyme, the deficiency of which promotes atherogenesis. This has been shown to be caused by GPX1 enzyme deficiencies, caused in turn by genetic deficiencies or errors[20]. Various neurodegenerative disorders (NDDs) have been associated with low levels of GSH all caused from GPX1 genetic errors, NDDs such as Alzheimer disease, Amyotrophic Lateral Sclerosis, Friedreich's Ataxia, Huntington's disease, Multiple Sclerosis, and Parkinson's disease. In addition, oxidative stress causing protein misfold may turn to other NDDs including: Creutzfeldt-Jakob disease, Bovine Spongiform Encephalopathy, Kuru,

Gerstmann-Straussler-Scheinker syndrome, and Fatal Familial Insomnia[21].

Autism As a Gentic Mitochondrial Disease

Mitochonrdrial disease (another genetic disorder) is felt to be the cause of autism or being on the AS, and there is always reduced or nil GSH in those patients. Think how much these patients might be able to benefit from a real workable GSH when it becomes available (another FDA approval we may need to go after? We have videos).

Toxins Such As Acetominophen

For decades emergency room doctors have known that too much acetaminophen (or APAP) can deplete your GSH levels and cause liver necrosis and death[22]. Typically, because they've not had a real, functional, workable GSH they've given NAC IV or orally – however they could get it in. The NAC (N-acetyl-cysteine or Cysteine) not only blocks acetaminophen absorption from the small bowel, but creates a GSH which protects the liver from toxicity[23]. It has saved thousands and thousands of lives (acetaminophen overdose is the #1 attempted cause of medication overdose suicide in the USA) but also tens of thousands have died horrible deaths related to the overdose because of lack of viable treatment options (i.e. GSH).

A newer understanding of acetaminophen toxicity and death has recently been shown to involve three processes – necroptosis, apoptosis, and a third programmed cell death, *ferroptosis*, is also involved in acetaminophen induced cell death in primary hepatocytes[24].

Summary

GSH deficiencies can be caused by genetic disorders, vitamin deficiencies (such as selenium and others), and toxin overdoses (such as acetaminophen and many others). There has been little to no option to deal with these conditions in the past – all leading to toxicity issues and other problems.

Chapter 7

Glutathione Foods – Do They Exist? Do They Work?

Let me just make a quick and simple list here – but some of these are obvious.

Glutamine containing foods: Eggs, beans (legumes) nuts, poultry, beef (especially liver), and fish/shellfish.

Cysteine containing foods: Soybeans, beef, lamb, sunflowers seeds, chicken, oats, pork, fish, cheese, eggs, and beans (legumes)[25].

Selenium containg foods: Brazillian nuts, Tuna, Halibut (cooked), Sardines (canned), Grass-fed beef, Turkey (boneless), Beef liver, Chicken, Eggs, and Spinach[26].

Alpha Lipoic Acid (ALA): "Various meat products, particularly organ meats such as the heart, liver and kidneys, and vegetables such as broccoli and spinach. ALA is also present in yeast, particularly brewer's yeast."[27]

Whey Protein: Hundreds of studies have shown how whey protein elevates GSH levels and decreases

GSSG levels (good job!). Here's the best, referenced here[28].

Ascorbic Acid (Vitamin C) containing foods: Citrus fruits, etc. even quercitin[29].

Liver: Is supposed to be a glutathione enhancer but I can find no research to support this contention.

Chapter 8

Glutathione IV/Injectable – Does It Work & Is It Worth It?

Reduced Intravenous (IV) or Injectable glutathione (GSH) sounds awesome in theory, doesn't it?

Here are the problems we've discovered:

- Air or oxygen has been inadvertently introduced into the tubing, bag, and syringe causing the GSH to be oxidized – the most common problem we found. The tubing and bags are not air proof either so that's a problem. We also think most pharmacies do not understand the need to keep the manufacturing performed in an anerobic (oxygen free) environment.

- Expense is a major hurdle for injectable or IV glutathione. This prevents access for many people.

- To obtain IV or injectable glutathione, a patient must see a physician who will prescribe it. Hmmm, first of all good luck with that – finding a doctor (MD or DO) who will write a prescription for IV or injectable glutathione. Next, good luck finding a pharmacy who fills it and manufactures it correctly. Third, the requirement of having to interface with a physician added a whole other level of expense.

So IV/injectable glutathione is of questionable efficacy, high expense and obtaining it is difficult at best.

There has to be a better option.

Chapter 9

FDA Level Product Development – It Has To Be THAT Good

In modern America, to take a product in front of the FDA for approval as a drug or as a supplement on which you desire to make drug claims (such as ours), it had better be real, because a lot of money is about to be spent in the process (anywhere from $30 million to $1 billion plus).

Actually it better be like *real effective*. As in functional. Validated. Absorbable. Reduced. Stable. Palatable.

But most of the IP (intellectual property) better be solid and undbreakable in order to protect the investors. The expense of taking a product through the three phases of FDA approval can easily run up to a billion dollars (for all the testing and proof of efficacy), but we determined that since our glutathione was GRAS/E and would be used topically, for the approval we wished to obtain (shingles treatement), the cost was estimated to be a paltry $30 million.

Shingles is the #1 cause of suicide in people over age 70 in the USA and Western Europe. It is horrible. And if you have it on your eyes or forehead it can be deadly or extremely debilitating. And the pain is endless and horrific.

Having the first functional working glutathione has taught us a few shocking things. Such as it seems to be pretty anti-viral. We just need to really prove that (so do not believe me, as we do not yet have adequate scientific proof) in order to legally say that – according to the FDA. So proving that point is where the $30 million will fall. Then the many other things we've discovered along the way.

(NOTE: You just can't go around making "medical claims" – as those are called – you need to have validation according to the very stringent FDA standards, and that, is ALWAYS a very expensive process.)

Chapter 10

My Glutathione Article Validating Our Product

Effects of a Novel Oral Glutathione Supplement in Liposome Suspension on Serum GSH and Systemic Oxidative Stress Biomarker GSSG in Humans

Stephen N. Pitcher

Dan Purser M.D.

<u>Abstract</u>

A novel liquid-based oral glutathione supplement was evaluated for serum GSH (reduced glutathione) and systemic oxidative stress biomarker GSSG (oxidized glutathione) levels in four human volunteers. The supplement was taken orally by three of the participants, and applied topically by one participant. Human serum GSH and GSSG levels were sampled initially before ingestion for baseline, and three times over eight hours after ingestion or application of the supplement. Also, the participants continued to take the supplement once every morning at least 30 minutes before meals for four weeks. The participants were sampled once each week during the four week study period to collect data for long-term effects.

Every participant experienced a short-term increase in serum GSH of at least thirty percent, and all participants demonstrated a long-term progressive reduction of oxidized glutathione GSSG of at least thirty percent. GSH and GSSG results were reported in absolute and ratiometric bar chart form. The ratio of GSH/GSSG is an important and well understood marker for cellular oxidative stress. The results indicated that the glutathione delivered by the supplement was bioavailable, unlike other pill and capsule delivery forms, and provided a long-term reduction in systemic cellular oxidative stress.

Introduction

Glutathione (GSH) is often referred to as the body's master antioxidant. Composed of three amino acids - cysteine, glycine, and glutamate - glutathione can be found in virtually every cell of the human body. The highest concentration of glutathione is in the liver, making it critical in the body's detoxification process.

Glutathione is also an essential component to the body's natural defense system. Viruses, bacteria, heavy metal toxicity, radiation, certain medications, and even the normal process of aging can all cause free-radical damage to healthy cells and deplete glutathione. Glutathione depletion has been correlated with lower immune function and increased vulnerability to infection due to the liver's reduced ability to detoxify. As the generation of free radicals exceeds the body's ability to neutralize and eliminate them, oxidative stress occurs. A primary function of glutathione is to alleviate this oxidative stress.

Biochemistry, Metabolism

Reduced glutathione (GSH) is a linear tripeptide of L-glutamine, L-cysteine, and glycine. Technically N-L-gamma-glutamyl-cysteinyl glycine or L-glutathione, the molecule has a sulfhydryl (SH) group on the cysteinyl portion, which accounts for its strong electron-donating character.

As electrons are lost, the molecule becomes oxidized, and two such molecules become linked (dimerized) by a disulfide bridge to form glutathione disulfide or oxidized glutathione (GSSG). This linkage is reversible upon re-reduction.

GSH is under tight homeostatic control both intracellularly and extracellularly. A dynamic balance is maintained between GSH synthesis, its recycling from GSSG/oxidized glutathione, and its utilization.

GSH synthesis involves two closely linked, enzymatically-controlled reactions that utilize ATP. First, cysteine and glutamate are combined by gamma-glutamyl cysteinyl synthetase. Second, GSH synthetase combines gamma-glutamylcysteine with glycine to generate GSH. As GSH levels rise, they self-limit further GSH synthesis; otherwise, cysteine availability is usually rate-limiting. Fasting, protein-energy malnutrition, or other dietary amino acid deficiencies limit GSH synthesis. GSH recycling is catalyzed by glutathione disulfide reductase, which uses reducing equivalents from NADPH to reconvert GSSG to 2GSH. The reducing power of ascorbate helps conserve systemic GSH.

GSH is used as a cofactor by (1) multiple peroxidase enzymes, to detoxify peroxides generated from oxygen radical attack on biological molecules; (2) transhydrogenases, to reduce oxidized centers on DNA, proteins, and other biomolecules; and (3) glutathione S-transferases (GST) to conjugate GSH with endogenous substances (e.g., estrogens), exogenous electrophiles (e.g., arene oxides, unsaturated carbonyls, organic halides), and diverse xenobiotics. Low GST activity may increase risk for disease—but paradoxically, some GSH conjugates can also be toxic.

Direct attack by free radicals and other oxidative agents can also deplete GSH. The homeostatic glutathione redox cycle attempts to keep GSH repleted as it is being consumed. Amounts available from foods are limited (less that 150 mg/day), and oxidative depletion can outpace synthesis.

The liver is the largest GSH reservoir. The parenchymal cells synthesize GSH for P450 conjugation and numerous other metabolic requirements—then export GSH as a systemic source of SH-reducing power. GSH is carried in the bile to the intestinal luminal compartment. Epithelial tissues of the kidney tubules, intestinal lining and lung have substantial P450 activity—and modest capacity to export GSH.

GSH equivalents circulate in the blood predominantly as cystine, the oxidized and more stable form of cysteine. Cells import cystine from the blood, reconvert it to cysteine (likely using ascorbate as cofactor), and from it synthesize GSH. Conversely, inside the cell, GSH helps re-reduce oxidized forms of other antioxidants—such as ascorbate and alpha-tocopherol.

Mechanism of Action

GSH is an extremely important cell protectant. It directly quenches reactive hydroxyl free radicals, other oxygen-centered free radicals, and radical centers on DNA and other biomolecules. GSH is a primary protectant of skin, lens, cornea, and retina against radiation damage and other biochemical foundations of P450 detoxification in the liver, kidneys, lungs, intestinal, epithelia and other organs.

GSH is the essential cofactor for many enzymes that require thiol-reducing equivalents, and helps keep redox-sensitive active sites on enzyme in the necessary reduced state. Higher-order thiol cell systems, the metallothioneins, thioredoxins and other redox regulator proteins are ultimately regulated by GSH levels—and the GSH/GSSG redox ratio. GSH/GSSG balance is crucial to homeostasis— stabilizing the cellular biomolecular spectrum, and facilitating cellular performance and survival.

GSH and its metabolites also interface with energetics and neurotransmitter syntheses through several prominent metabolic pathways. GSH availability down-regulates the pro-inflammatory potential of leukotrienes and other eicosanoids. Recently discovered S-nitroso metabolites, generated in vivo from GSH and NO (nitric oxide), further diversify GSH's impact on metabolism.

Experimental Procedure

Four persons, one male and three females ranging in age from 23 to 83 years old agreed to participate. Each participant was assigned a number from #1 to #4:

Participant   Age

#1 Female   61 years old

#2 Male   55 years old

#3 Female   23 years old

#4 Female   83 years old

Supplement Formulation The supplement consisted of a 99.9% reduced glutathione (GSH) powder solubilized in a novel deoxygenated water and encapsulated in a plant-based phospholipid liposome structure using a proprietary method. A small amount of stevia and natural lemon and peppermint essential oil flavor was added. The effective dose of each supplementation was 550mg GSH/4g solution. The supplement was packaged in an airless dispenser to protect it from oxygen degradation.

Short Term Evaluation Participants were allowed to eat the morning of first collection, but refrained from taking antioxidant dietary supplements during the course of the four-week study period. The participants' blood was collected for baseline measurements at approximately 8AM by veinous puncture, the serum extracted, processed and frozen for later analysis. After collection, the participants immediately consumed the supplement by dispensing

4ml of the supplement formulation into their mouth and swished for 15-20 seconds and swallowed. They refrained from drinking for at least 15 minutes afterwards. The participant who used the product topically applied approximately the same amount onto the abdomen and soft areas under the arms. Blood samples were collected again at 2hrs, 6hrs, and 8hrs after first collection.

Long Term Evaluation The participants consumed the supplement one time per day in the morning for a 4 week period. Participants' blood was collected each week at exactly 7 day intervals for 4 weeks at approximately 10 AM. Participants were instructed to consume the supplement 4 hours prior to collection. The serum was extracted, processed and frozen for later analysis. All samples were assayed within 30 days of collection.

Analysis GSH and GSSG serum levels were assayed using the BioVision (Milpitas, Ca) Glutathione Fluorometric Assay Kit (GSH, GSSG, and Total) k264. Wasatch Scientific Laboratories (Murray, Ut) was contracted to perform the assay using the BioVision fluorometric kit and method.

Whole blood samples were collected and immediately centrifuged to separate the serum from the red blood cells and heavier components. Approximately 120µl of serum was added to 40µl of an ice-cold proprietary perchloric acid PCA buffer in a 1ml aliquot, vortexed, and stored on ice for 5 minutes. Then the mixture was centrifuged at 13,000G for 2 minutes, and the supernatant was collected and frozen at -60degC.

The assay for the Short Term Test (first test) and Long-Term Test (second test) utilized their own separate BioVision Glutathione Fluorometric Assay Kit. A standard curve for GSH and GSSG was created, and then the prepared serum samples were tested at two different dilutions to determine the optimal dilution for the best dynamic resolution of the assay. Then samples were processed and assayed in duplicate pairs at the chosen dilution. The results of each pair were reviewed and compared for repeatability and best-fit samples were used.

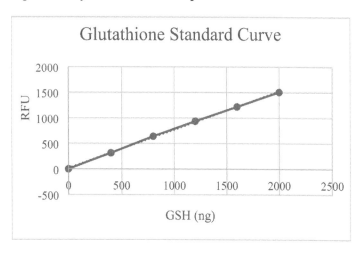

Fig. 1 GSH Standard Curve (Short-Term analysis)

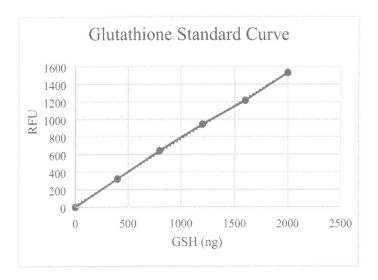

Fig. 2 GSH Standard Curve (Long-Term analysis)

Results

The results of two separate assays, Short-Term Test and Long-Term Test, were compiled and displayed in tabular and graphical form in an Excel spreadsheet. In addition, ratiometric results of GSH/GSSG were created for each sample.

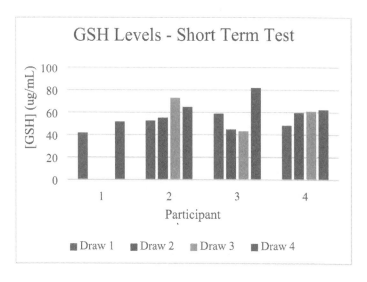

Fig. 3 GSH Levels Short-Term Test

Draw 1 = Baseline (B)

Draw 2 = B+4 hours

Draw 3 = B+6 hours

Draw 4 = B+8 hours

Short-Term Test Results

All participants in the Short-Term Test experienced an increase in serum GSH levels that appeared to peak approximately 6-8 hours after ingestion. The GSH increase was on average 30% above baseline levels.

Participant #1 a female, applied the supplement topically and still experienced elevated GSH serum levels. This participant was not assayed at Draw 2 and 3 because of limitations of the number of sample wells in the initial assay, due to first run dilution test requirements.

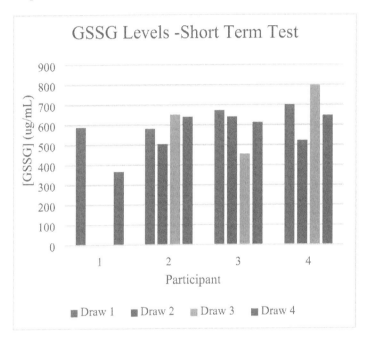

Fig. 4 GSSG Levels Short-Term Test

Note that GSSG levels in the Short-Term Test reported in Fig. 4 above, appeared to respond differently for each participant. The most significant change was an almost 50% reduction in participant #1 who applied the supplement topically. In participants

#3 and #4, the GSSG levels on average reduced slightly from baseline.

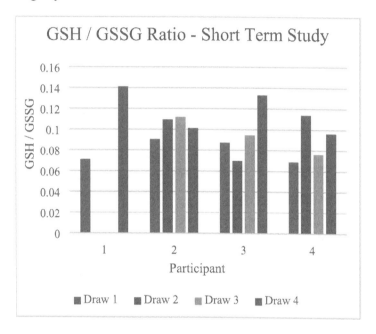

Fig. 5 GSH/GSSG Ratio – Short Term Study

However, Fig. 5 above showing the ratio of GSH/GSSG remarkably shows that the supplement provided a short-term antioxidant benefit. The GSH/GSSG redox ratio is an accepted standard to measure cellular oxidative stress. For this study, the most important feature is the redox ratio trend over time. After ingestion, every participant experienced an increase in the redox ratio compared to baseline, even after more then 8 hours after consuming or applying the supplement.

Long-Term Test Results

The Long-Term Test was designed to determine if a lasting or cumulative benefit of supplementation was evident. Once a week, immediately after the Short-Term Test for 4 weeks the participants were sampled, and human serum GSH and GSSG was assayed at the end of the trial. Samples were collected at the same time of day at 10AM for each blood draw. Note that Draw #1 – Week 1 results were not shown, due to an accidental thaw of the samples causing GSH oxidation.

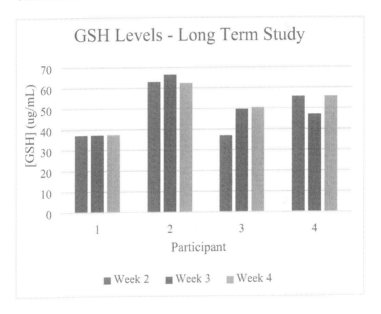

Fig. 6 GSH Levels – Long Term Study

Participants' GSH serum levels which are displayed above show mixed results. Participants #1 and #3 GSH levels are very close to their study baseline levels with no significant increase. Participants #2 and #4 produced a long-term increase of approximately 20-22%. Long-Term serum GSH levels when viewed alone showed positive results in in both of these participants, but unremarkable for participants #1 and #3. However, more importantly their GSSG levels indicated an important trend for all of the participants as demonstrated in figure 7 below.

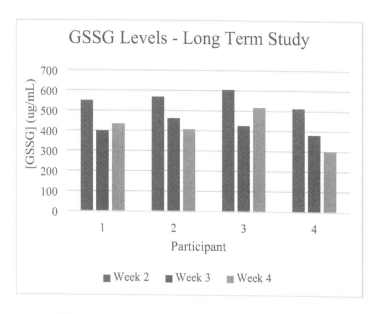

Fig. 7 GSSG Levels – Long Term Study

As shown in the figure above, all participants experienced a decrease in long-term oxidized GSSG serum levels. GSH is oxidized inside cells and converted to GSSG. Then a portion of the GSSG is shuttled out of the cells, into the intracellular space and into the blood. When the GSH/GSSG redox ratio is calculated, a true reduction in cellular oxidation is evident.

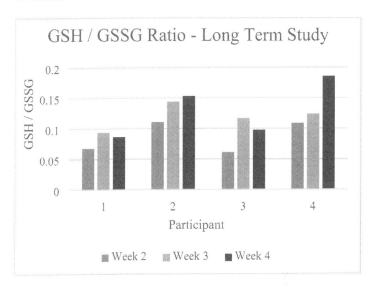

Fig. 8 GSH/GSSG Ratio – Long Term Study

The GSH/GSSG redox ratio increased for all participants indicating a sustained and cumulative decrease in cellular oxidative stress. It is interesting to note that participants #3 and #4 represent a wide age and health gap, female 23 years and healthy vs. female 83 years with health issues due to age respectively.

The supplement had a positive long-term effect in both young and old, with the older participants experiencing a greater rise in the redox ratio. Also, the data shows that participant #1 received a redox benefit, even by applying the product topically. It should be mentioned that this participant only applied about one third of the dose compared to the oral participants, not following specific dosing instructions. The results for all of the participants clearly show the benefits of the novel glutathione supplement as seen in the GSH/GSSG redox ratio.

Figure 9 below displays the GSH/GSSG ratio that has been normalized to the participant's baseline levels. This figure gives a truer comparison of the change in redox over time as a result of supplementation of the test product.

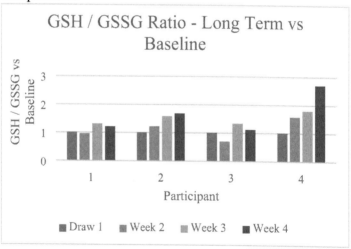

Fig. 9 GSH/GSSG Ratio – Long Term vs. Baseline

This figure reveals some interesting results. All participants had a net average increase above baseline redox ratio, with participants #2 (Male 55 years) and #4 (female 83 years) showing the greatest increase. It is anticipated that participant #1 (female 61 years) would have produced a higher result if the dosage requirements were followed more consistently.

Conclusion

The effects of the novel glutathione supplementation indicated a bioavailability of reduced glutathione and its' short-term and long-term effects as indicated in the serum concentrations of reduced glutathione GSH and oxidized glutathione GSSG. All participants produced a noticeable increase in GSH/GSSG redox ratio indicating a true reduction in cellular oxidative stress, with the older participants (age 55 – 83) producing higher ratios. This may be consistent with an assumption that the older participants may have had greater cellular oxidative stress to be reduced. However, it is interesting to note that the older participants (55 years +, excluding younger participant #3) had higher redox ratios at baseline.

The results of this study are particularly encouraging compared to a more comprehensive oral glutathione study[1] published in the Journal of Alternative and

Complementary Medicine In 2011. This randomized, double blind, placebo controlled study administered 500mg 2X per day of reduced glutathione orally in capsule form to human participants. It measured GSH, GSSG, total glutathione, and two other inflammation marker assays. The study reported no antioxidant effects, no increase in GSH or decrease in GSSG, or reduction in measured inflammatory markers. It is interesting that the oral dose of reduced glutathione in that study was almost twice of the current study.

A greater statistical confidence in the results in the current study can be achieved if it is repeated with a greater number of participants and introducing placebo control. Another recommendation is to include other means of measuring oxidative stress and inflammation such as urinary Hydroxyde-xoyguanosine (8-OHdG) and urinary F2 isoprostanes (F2-isoP) assays.

[1] Allen, Jason and Ryan, Bradley D., *Effects of Oral Glutathione Supplementation on Systemic Oxidative Stress Biomarkers in Human Volunteers*. J Altern Complement Med. 2011 Sep; 17(9): 827–833.

Chapter 11

Key Glutathione Studies & Articles

Some Key Glutathione Articles

The following are some of my favorie articles on glutathione. I hope they help and give you some ideas.

N Am J Med Sci. 2013 Mar;5(3):213-9. doi: 10.4103/1947-2714.109193.

Antioxidant Enzymes and Lipid Peroxidation in Type 2 Diabetes Mellitus Patients with and without Nephropathy.

Kumawat M[1], Sharma TK, Singh I, Singh N, Ghalaut VS, Vardey SK, Shankar V.

Author information

• [1]Department of Biochemistry, Pandit Bhagwat Dayal Sharma University of Health Sciences, Post Graduate Institute of Medical Sciences, Rohtak, Haryana, India.

Abstract

BACKGROUND:

Oxidative stress has been considered to be a pathogenic factor of diabetic complications including nephropathy. There are many controversies and limited studies regarding the antioxidant enzymes in diabetic nephropathy.

AIM:

This study was to evaluate the levels of antioxidant enzymes and lipid peroxidation in Type-2 Diabetes Mellitus (DM) patients with and without nephropathy.

MATERIALS AND METHODS:

The study included 90 age and sex matched subjects. Blood samples of all subjects were analyzed for all biochemical and oxidative stress parameters.

RESULTS:

The malondialdehyde (MDA) levels and catalase (CAT) activity were significantly increased and reduced glutathione (GSH) levels and activities of glutathione peroxidase (GPx) and glutathione reductase (GR) were significantly decreased in Type-2 DM with and without nephropathy as compared to controls and also in Type-2 DM with nephropathy as compared to Type-2 DM without nephropathy. There were an excellent positive correlation of glycohemoglobin (HbA1c) with MDA and a good negative correlation of GPx with GSH in controls. There were positive correlations of GR, CAT, and superoxide dismutase (SOD) with MDA in Type-2 diabetes patients with nephropathy.

CONCLUSIONS:

Intensity of oxidative stress in Type-2 diabetic patients with nephropathy is greater when compared with Type-2 diabetic patients without nephropathy as compared to the controls.

KEYWORDS:

Antioxidant enzymes; Glycosylated hemoglobin and diabetic nephropathy; Lipid profile; Malondialdehyde; Non-insulin dependent diabetes mellitus; Reduced glutathione

PMID: 23626958 PMCID:PMC3632026 DOI: 10.4103/1947-2714.109193   Redox   Biol. 2016   Oct;9:220-228.   doi: 10.1016/j.redox.2016.08.012. Epub 2016 Aug 21.

Quercetin affects glutathione levels and redox ratio in human aortic endothelial cells not through oxidation but formation and cellular export of quercetin-glutathione conjugates and upregulation of glutamate-cysteine ligase.

Li C[1], Zhang WJ[1], Choi J[1], Frei B[2].

Author information

Abstract

Endothelial dysfunction due to vascular inflammation and oxidative stress critically contributes to the etiology of atherosclerosis. The intracellular redox environment plays a key role in regulating endothelial cell function and is intimately linked to cellular thiol status, including and foremost glutathione (GSH). In the present study we investigated whether and how the dietary flavonoid, quercetin, affects GSH status of human aortic endothelial cells (HAEC) and their response to oxidative stress. We found that treating cells with buthionine sulfoximine to deplete cellular GSH levels significantly reduced the capacity of quercetin to inhibit lipopolysaccharide (LPS)-induced oxidant production. Furthermore, incubation of HAEC with quercetin caused a transient decrease and then full recovery of cellular GSH concentrations. The initial decline in GSH was not accompanied by a corresponding increase in glutathione disulfide (GSSG). To the contrary, GSSG levels, which were less than 0.5% of GSH levels at baseline (0.26 ± 0.01 vs. 64.7 ± 1.9 nmol/mg protein, respectively), decreased by about 25% during incubation with quercetin. As a result, the GSH: GSSG ratio increased by about 70%, from 253±7 to 372±23. These quercetin-induced changes in GSH and GSSG levels were not affected by treating HAEC with 500µM ascorbic acid phosphate for 24h to increase intracellular ascorbate levels. Incubation of HAEC with quercetin also led to the appearance of extracellular quercetin-glutathione conjugates, which was paralleled by upregulation of the multidrug resistance protein 1 (MRP1). Furthermore, quercetin slightly but significantly increased mRNA and protein levels of glutamate-cysteine ligase (GCL) catalytic and modifier subunits. Taken together, our results suggest that quercetin causes loss of GSH in HAEC, not because of oxidation but due to formation and cellular export of quercetin-glutathione conjugates. Induction by quercetin of GCL subsequently restores GSH levels, thereby suppressing LPS-induced oxidant production.

KEYWORDS:

Endothelial cells; Glutathione; Oxidants; Quercetin

PMID: 27572418 PMCID: PMC5011167 DOI: 10.1016/j.redox.2016.08.012

Oxid Med Cell Longev. 2016;2016:6585737. doi: 10.1155/2016/6585737. Epub 2016 Mar 31.

Antioxidant Effects of Sheep Whey Protein on Endothelial Cells.

Kerasioti   E[1], Stagos   D[1], Georgatzi   V[1], Bregou E[1], Priftis A[1], Kafantaris I[1], Kouretas D[1].

Author information

Abstract
Excessive production of reactive oxygen species (ROS) may cause endothelial dysfunction and consequently vascular disease. In the present study, the possible protective effects of sheep whey protein (SWP) from tert-butyl hydroperoxide- (tBHP-) induced oxidative stress in endothelial cells (EA.hy926) were assessed using oxidative stress biomarkers. These oxidative stress biomarkers were glutathione (GSH) and ROS levels determined by flow cytometry. Moreover, thiobarbituric acid-reactive substances (TBARS), protein carbonyls (CARB), and oxidized glutathione (GSSG) were determined spectrophotometrically. The results showed that SWP at 0.78, 1.56, 3.12, and 6.24 mg of protein mL(-1) increased GSH up to 141%, while it decreased GSSG to 46.7%, ROS to 58.5%, TBARS to 52.5%, and CARB to 49.0%. In conclusion, the present study demonstrated for the first time that SWP protected endothelial cells from oxidative stress. Thus, SWP may be used for developing food supplements or biofunctional foods to attenuate vascular disturbances associated with oxidative stress.

PMID: 27127549   PMCID: PMC4830741   DOI: 10.1155/2016/6585737

Can J Physiol Pharmacol. 1985 May;63(5):431-7.

Postabsorption antidotal effects of N-acetylcysteine on acetaminophen-induced hepatotoxicity in the mouse.

Whitehouse LW, Wong LT, Paul CJ, Pakuts A, Solomonraj G.

Abstract

Male Swiss Webster mice, treated with N-acetylcysteine (NAC, 500 mg/kg po) 1 h following acetaminophen (NAPA, 350 mg/kg po) administration, had control levels of transaminases indicating that NAC protects against NAPA-induced hepatotoxicity by postabsorption antidotal mechanism(s). Hepatic congestion induced by NAPA was reduced by NAC. Significantly higher elimination rate constants (K) for indocyanine green (500 micrograms/kg, iv) in mice treated with NAPA and NAC (K = 0.676 +/- 0.062) than in animals receiving NAPA alone (0.341 +/- 0.105) suggested NAC improved or preserved the hepatic circulation of the compromised liver. This NAC-induced improvement and (or) preservation of hepatic circulation was reflected in biliary and urinary excretion of acetaminophen and its metabolites by a general increase in elimination during the first 6 h (70.2 +/- 2.6 vs. 32.6 +/- 7.1%), and in the repletion of glutathione (GSH) in the liver by a return to control levels more quickly (3 vs. greater than 5 h) following depletion by NAPA. The metabolic consequences of the postabsorption antidotal effect of NAC in the compromised liver was a preferential excretion of sulphydryl-derived metabolites in the 1-4 h bile (GSH conjugate 11.30 +/- 1.25 vs. 7.25 +/- 0.39%) which was subsequently observed in the urine by preferential excretion of glutathione degradation products.

PMID: 4041986 <u>Am Fam Physician.</u> 1980 Jul;22(1):83-7.

Acetaminophen hepatotoxicity and overdose.

Bailey BO.

Abstract
Acetaminophen is a widely available and frequently recommended over-the-counter analgesic and antipyretic. Chronic doses in excess of 5 Gm. per day and acute doses of as little as 7 Gm. have caused hepatic damage in adults. Larger doses may be fatal. The hepatotoxicity, which is due to metabolic transformation of the acetaminophen to an alkylating agent, can be palliated or avoided by prompt treatment. Blood levels over 200 micrrograms per mL. four hours after ingestion correlate with severe hepatotoxicity. Clinical trials have shown N-acetylcysteine (NAC) to be a specific antidote when administered within eight hours of an acute ingestion.

PMID: 7386356 `Kardon T, Mandl J, Szarka A.

Author information
Abstract
The recently described form of programmed cell death, ferroptosis can be induced by agents causing GSH depletion or the inhibition of GPX4. Ferroptosis clearly shows distinct morphologic, biochemical and genetic features from apoptosis, necrosis and autophagy. Since NAPQI the highly reactive metabolite of the widely applied analgesic and antipyretic, acetaminophen induces a cell death

which can be characterized by GSH depletion, GPX inhibition and caspase independency the involvement of ferroptosis in acetaminophen induced cell death has been investigated. The specific ferroptosis inhibitor ferrostatin-1 failed to elevate the viability of acetaminophen treated HepG2 cells. It should be noticed that these cells do not form NAPQI due to the lack of phase I enzyme expression therefore GSH depletion cannot be observed. However in the case of acetaminophen treated primary mouse hepatocytes the significant elevation of cell viability could be observed upon ferrostatin-1 treatment. Similar to ferrostatin-1 treatment, the addition of the RIP1 kinase inhibitor necrostatin-1 could also elevate the viability of acetaminophen treated primary hepatocytes. Ferrostatin-1 has no influence on the expression of CYP2E1 or on the cellular GSH level which suggest that the protective effect of ferrostatin-1 in APAP induced cell death is not based on the reduced metabolism of APAP to NAPQI or on altered NAPQI conjugation by cellular GSH. Our results suggest that beyond necroptosis and apoptosis a third programmed cell death, ferroptosis is also involved in acetaminophen induced cell death in primary hepatocytes.

PMID: 25962350 DOI: 10.1007/s12253-015-9946-3

Scand J Clin Lab Invest. 2012 Apr;72(2):152-7. doi: 10.3109/00365513.2011.646299. Epub 2012 Jan 2.

Plasma thiol status is altered in children with mitochondrial diseases.

Salmi H[1], Leonard JV, Rahman S, Lapatto R.

Author information

Abstract

OBJECTIVE:

This study was undertaken to investigate thiol metabolism as a marker of oxidative stress and antioxidative defence capacity in a cohort of children with biochemically and/or genetically confirmed mitochondrial disease. Previous studies suggest that lower glutathione levels, which have been shown to further compromise mitochondrial function, may occur in these diseases. Better understanding of the pathogenesis of mitochondrial diseases is important in order to improve their treatment.

METHODS:

We studied plasma and erythrocyte glutathione and cysteine levels, the activities of erythrocyte glutathione peroxidase (GPx), glutathione reductase (GR), glucose 6-phosphate dehydrogenase G6PDH) and glutathione S-transferase (GST), as well as the levels of erythrocyte thiobarbituric acid-reactive species (TBA-RS) and protein carbonyls in 10 children with a biochemical and/or genetic diagnosis of mitochondrial disease and six controls.

RESULTS:

Levels of reduced cysteine (CYSH) as well as reduced to oxidised cysteine ratio were lower in plasma of patients with mitochondrial diseases ($p = 0.008$ and $p = 0.02$, respectively). Plasma levels of reduced glutathione (GSH) were low in patients with mitochondrial diseases, mostly below the detection limit. We did not detect significant differences in erythrocyte thiols or glutathione-related enzyme activities.

CONCLUSION:

Plasma thiols and their redox state are altered in patients with mitochondrial diseases, suggesting an increase in oxidative stress and depletion of antioxidant supplies. If confirmed in further studies, this relative thiol deficiency could be an important factor in the pathophysiology of mitochondrial diseases.

PMID: 22208644 DOI: 10.3109/00365513.2011.646299

Neurol Res. 2017 Jan;39(1):73-82. Epub 2016 Nov 3.

Oxidative stress and mitochondrial dysfunction-linked neurodegenerative disorders.

Islam MT[1,2].

Author information

Abstract

Reactive species play an important role in physiological functions. Overproduction of reactive species, notably reactive oxygen (ROS) and nitrogen (RNS) species along with the failure of balance by the body's antioxidant enzyme systems results in destruction of cellular structures, lipids, proteins, and genetic materials such as DNA and RNA. Moreover, the effects of reactive species on mitochondria and their metabolic processes eventually cause a rise in ROS/RNS levels, leading to oxidation of mitochondrial proteins, lipids, and DNA. Oxidative stress has been considered to be linked to the etiology of many diseases, including neurodegenerative diseases (NDDs) such as Alzheimer diseases, Amyotrophic lateral sclerosis, Friedreich's ataxia, Huntington's disease, Multiple sclerosis, and Parkinson's diseases. In addition, oxidative stress causing protein misfold may turn to other NDDs include Creutzfeldt-Jakob disease, Bovine Spongiform Encephalopathy, Kuru, Gerstmann-Straussler-Scheinker syndrome, and Fatal Familial Insomnia. An overview of the oxidative stress and mitochondrial dysfunction-linked NDDs has been summarized in this review.

KEYWORDS:

AD: Alzheimer's disease; ALS: Amyotrophic lateral sclerosis; AP-1: activator protein 1; APP: Aβ precursor protein; Aβ: amyloid-β; BBB: blood–brain barrier; BER: base excision repair; BSE: Bovine Spongiform Encephalopathy; CAA: cerebral amyloid angiopathy; CAT: catalase; CBF: cerebral blood flow; CJD: Creutzfeldt-Jakob disease; CNS: central nervous system; COX: cyclooxygenase; CRP: C-reactive protein; Cyt-c: cytochrome c; DA: dopamine; DAG: diacylglycerol; DJ-1: protein deglycase 1; DNMT: DNA methyltransferase; DOPAC: 3, 4-dihydroxyphenylacetic acid; DRG: dorsal root ganglia; DSBs: double strand breaks; EPCs: endothelial progenitor cells; FFI: Fatal Familial Insomnia; FRDA: Friedreich's ataxia; GPx: glutathione peroxidase; GSH: glutathione; GSS: Gerstmann-Straussler-Scheinker syndrome; HD: Huntington's disease; HIF-1α: hypoxia-inducible factor-1 alpha; HNE: 4- hydroxynonenal; HVA: homovanillic acid; IL: interleukin; IR: ionizing radiation; JAK: Janus kinase; MAO-B: monoamine oxidase B; MDA: malondialdehyde; MMPs: matrix metalloproteins; NADP: nicotinamide adenine dinucleotide phosphate; NDDs: neurodegenerative diseases; NF-κB: nuclear factor kappa B; NFTs:

neurofibrillary tangles; NHEJ: non-homologous end joining; NHR: nucleotide excision repair; Neurodegenerative diseases; PD: Parkinson's disease; PG: prostaglandin; PGC-1α: peroxisome proliferator-activated receptor-γ co-activator-1α; PPL: phospholipase; PrP: prion protein; RNS: reactive nitrogen species; ROS: reactive oxygen species; SC: spinal cord; SMCs: smooth muscle cells; SOD: superoxide dismutase; SSBs: single strand breaks; TGF-β: tumor growth factor-beta; TNF-α: tumor necrosis factor-alpha; TOMM40: a gene associated with AD; TSEs: Transmissible Spongiform Encephalopathies; VEGF: vascular endothelial growth factor; iNOS: inducible nitric oxide synthase; mitochondrial dysfunction; mtDNA: mitochondrial DNA; mtMP: mitochondrial membrane permeability/potential; oxidative stress

PMID: 27809706 DOI: 10.1080/01616412.2016.1251711

Br J Haematol. 1964 Oct;10:477-84.

GLUTATHIONE CONCENTRATION AND STABILITY IN THE RED BLOOD CELLS IN VARIOUS DISEASE STATES, AND SOME OBSERVATIONS ON THE MECHANISM OF ACTION OF ACETYL-PHENYLHYDRAZINE.

SABINE JC. PMID: 14221774

Is glutamine a conditionally essential amino acid?

Lacey JM[1], Wilmore DW.

Author information

Abstract

The nonessential amino acid glutamine has recently been the focus of extensive scientific interest because of its importance in cell and tissue cultures and its physiologic role in animals and humans. Glutamine appears to be a unique amino acid, serving as a preferred respiratory fuel for rapidly proliferating cells, such as enterocytes and lymphocytes; a regulator of acid-base balance through the production of urinary ammonia; a carrier of nitrogen between tissues; and an important precursor of nucleic acids, nucleotides, amino sugars, and proteins. Abundant evidence suggests that glutamine may become a "conditionally essential" amino acid in the critically ill. During stress the body's requirements for glutamine appear to exceed the individual's ability to produce sufficient amounts of this amino acid. Provision of supplemental glutamine in specialized enteral or parenteral feeding may enhance nutritional management and augment recovery of the seriously ill while minimizing hospital stay.

PMID: 2080048

J Biol Chem. 1975 Feb 25;250(4):1422-6.

Regulation of gamma-glutamyl-cysteine synthetase by nonallosteric feedback inhibition by glutathione.

Richman PG, Meister A.

Abstract

Gamma-Glutamyl-cysteine synthetase is inhibited by glutathione under conditions similar to those which prevail in vivo, thus strongly suggesting a physiologically significant feedback mechanism. Inhibition by glutathione, which is not allosteric, appears to involve the binding of glutathione to the glutamate site of the enzyme as well as to another enzyme site; the latter binding appears to require a sulfhydryl group since ophthalmic acid (gamma-glutamyl-alpha-aminobutyryl-glycine) is only a weak inhibitor. The finding that glutathione regulates its own synthesis by inhibiting synthesis of gamma-glutamyl-cysteine appears to explain observations on patients with 5-oxoprolinuria, who were shown to have a block in the gamma-glutamyl cycle consisting of a marked deficiency of glutathione synthetase and consequently of glutathione. These patients produce greater than normal amounts of gamma-glutamyl-cysteine, which is converted by the action of gamma-glutamyl cyclotransferase to 5-oxoproline; production of the latter compound exceeds the capacity of 5-oxoprolinase to convert it to glutamate. The apparent Km value for L-cysteine for gamma-glutamyl-cysteine synthetase (0.35 mM) is not far from **intracellular concentrations of L-cysteine suggesting that the availability of L-cysteine may also play a role in the regulation of glutathione synthesis**.

PMID:1112810

Front Pharmacol. 2014 Apr 11;5:73. doi: 10.3389/fphar.2014.00073. eCollection 2014.

Glutathione synthesis is compromised in erythrocytes from individuals with HIV.

Morris D[1], Ly J[1], Chi PT[2], Daliva J[2], Nguyen T[2], Soofer C[2], Chen YC[2], Lagman M[2], Venketaraman V[1].

Author information
Abstract

We demonstrated that the levels of enzymes responsible for the synthesis of glutathione (GSH) such as glutathione synthase (GSS), glutamate-cysteine ligase-catalytic subunit (GCLC), and glutathione reductase (GSR) were significantly reduced in the red blood cells (RBCs) isolated from individuals with human immunodeficiency virus (HIV) infection and this reduction correlated with decreased levels of intracellular GSH. GSH content in RBCs can be used as a marker for increased overall oxidative stress and immune dysfunctions caused by HIV infection. Our data supports our hypothesis that compromised levels of GSH in HIV infected individuals' is due to decreased levels of GSH-synthetic enzymes. The role of GSH in combating oxidative stress and improving the functions of immune cells in HIV patients' indicates the benefit of an antioxidant supplement which can reduce the cellular damage and promote the functions of immune cells.

KEYWORDS:

GCL; GSR; GSS; HIV; glutathione

PMID: 24782776 PMCID: PMC3990052 DOI: 10.3389/fphar.2014.00073

BBA Clin. 2016 May 29;6:38-44. doi: 10.1016/j.bbacli.2016.05.006. eCollection 2016.

Analysis of glutathione levels in the brain tissue samples from HIV-1-positive individuals and subject with Alzheimer's disease and its implication in the pathophysiology of the disease process.

Saing   T[1], Lagman   M[1], Castrillon   J[2], Gutierrez E[2], Guilford FT[3], Venketaraman V[2].

Author information

Abstract

HIV-1 positive individuals are at high risk for susceptibility to both pulmonary tuberculosis (TB) and extra-pulmonary TB, including TB meningitis (TBM) which is an extreme form of TB. The goals of this study are to determine the mechanisms responsible for compromised levels of glutathione (GSH) in the brain tissue samples derived from HIV-1-infected individuals and individuals with Alzheimer's disease (AD), investigate the possible underlying mechanisms responsible for GSH deficiency in these pathological conditions, and establish a link between GSH levels and pathophysiology of the disease processes. We demonstrated in the autopsied human brain tissues that the levels of total and reduced forms of GSH were significantly compromised in HIV-1 infected individuals compared to in healthy subjects and individuals with AD. Brain tissue samples derived from HIV-1-positive individuals had substantially higher levels of free radicals than that derived from healthy and AD individuals. Enzymes that are responsible for the de novo synthesis of GSH such as γ-glutamate cysteine-ligase catalytic subunit (GCLC-rate limiting step enzyme) and glutathione synthetase (GSS-enzyme involved in the second step reaction) were significantly decreased in the brain tissue samples derived from HIV-1-positive individuals with low CD4 + T-cells (< 200 cells/mm(3)) compared to healthy and AD individuals. Levels of glutathione reductase (GSR) were also decreased in the brain tissue samples derived from HIV-1 infected individuals. Overall, our findings demonstrate causes for GSH deficiency in the brain tissue from HIV-1 infected individuals explaining the possible reasons for increased susceptibility to the most severe form of extra-pulmonary TB, TBM.

KEYWORDS:

Glutathione; HIV; Opportunistic infections; Oxidative stress

PMID: 27335804

PMCID: PMC4908271

DOI: 10.1016/j.bbacli.2016.05.006

J Nutr. 2008 Oct;138(10):2025S-2031S.

Nonnutritive effects of glutamine.

Roth E[1].

Author information

Abstract

Glutamine is the most abundant free amino acid of the human body. Besides its role as a constituent of proteins and its importance in amino acid transamination, glutamine has regulatory capacity in immune and cell modulation. Glutamine deprivation reduces proliferation of lymphocytes, influences expression of surface activation markers on lymphocytes and monocytes, affects the production of cytokines, and stimulates apoptosis. Moreover, glutamine administration seems to have a positive effect on glucose metabolism in the state of insulin resistance. Glutamine influences a variety of different molecular pathways. Glutamine stimulates the formation of heat shock protein 70 in monocytes by enhancing the stability of mRNA, **influences the redox potential of the cell by enhancing the formation of glutathione**, induces cellular anabolic effects by increasing the cell volume, activates mitogen-activated protein kinases, and interacts with particular aminoacyl-transfer RNA synthetases in specific glutamine-sensing metabolism. Glutamine is applied under clinical conditions as an oral, parenteral, or enteral supplement either as the single amino acid or in the form of glutamine-containing dipeptides for preventing mucositis/stomatitis and for preventing glutamine-deficiency in critically ill patients. Because of the high turnover rate of glutamine, even high amounts of glutamine up to a daily administration of 30 g can be given without any important side effects.

PMID: 18806119

[PubMed - indexed for MEDLINE] J Interferon Cytokine Res. 2015 Nov;35(11):875-87. doi: 10.1089/jir.2014.0210. Epub 2015 Jul 2.

Liposomal Glutathione Supplementation Restores TH1 Cytokine Response to Mycobacterium tuberculosis Infection in HIV-Infected Individuals.

Ly J[1,2], Lagman M[1,2], Saing T[1], Singh MK[1,2], Tudela EV[1,2], Morris D[2], Anderson J[2], Daliva J[2], Ochoa C[3], Patel N[3], Pearce D[4], Venketaraman V[1,2].

Author information

Abstract

Cytokines are signaling biomolecules that serve as key regulators of our immune system. CD4(+) T-cells can be grouped into 2 major categories based on their cytokine profile: T-helper 1 (TH1) subset and T-helper 2 (TH2) subset. Protective immunity against HIV infection requires TH1-directed CD4 T-cell responses, mediated by cytokines, such as interleukin-1β (IL-1β), IL-12, interferon-γ (IFN-γ), and tumor necrosis factor-α (TNF-α). Cytokines released by the TH1 subset of CD4 T-cells are considered important for mediating effective immune responses against intracellular pathogens such as Mycobacterium tuberculosis (M. tb). Oxidative stress and redox imbalance that occur during HIV infection often lead to inappropriate immune responses. Glutathione (GSH) is an antioxidant present in nearly all cells and is recognized for its function in maintaining redox homeostasis. **Our laboratory previously reported that individuals**

with HIV infection have lower levels of GSH. In this study, we report a link between lower levels of GSH and dysregulation of TH1- and TH2-associated cytokines in the plasma samples of HIV-positive subjects. Furthermore, we demonstrate that supplementing individuals with HIV infection for 13 weeks with liposomal GSH (lGSH) resulted in a significant increase in the levels of TH1 cytokines, IL-1β, IL-12, IFN-γ, and TNF-α. lGSH supplementation in individuals with HIV infection also resulted in a substantial decrease in the levels of free radicals and immunosuppressive cytokines, IL-10 and TGF-β, relative to those in a placebo-controlled cohort. Finally, we determined the effects of lGSH supplementation in improving the functions of immune cells to control M. tb infection by conducting in vitro assays using peripheral blood mononuclear cells collected from HIV-positive individuals at post-GSH supplementation. **Our studies establish a correlation between low levels of GSH and increased susceptibility to M. tb infection through TH2-directed response, which may be relieved with lGSH supplementation enhancing the TH1 response.**

PMID: 26133750 PMCID: PMC4642835 DOI: 10.1089/jir.2014.0210

PLoS One. 2015 Mar 19;10(3):e0118436. doi: 10.1371/journal.pone.0118436. eCollection 2015.

Investigating the causes for decreased levels of glutathione in individuals with type II diabetes.

Lagman M[1], Ly J[2], Saing T[3], Kaur Singh M[1], Vera Tudela E[1], Morris D[2], Chi PT[1], Ochoa C[4], Sathananthan A[4], Venketaraman V[1].

Author information

Abstract

Tuberculosis (TB) remains an eminent global burden with one third of the world's population latently infected with Mycobacterium tuberculosis (M. tb). Individuals with compromised immune systems are especially vulnerable to M. tb infection. In fact, individuals with Type 2 Diabetes Mellitus (T2DM) are two to three times more susceptible to TB than those without T2DM. In this study, we report that individuals with T2DM have lower levels of glutathione (GSH) due to compromised levels of GSH synthesis and metabolism enzymes. Transforming growth factor beta (TGF-β), a cytokine that is known to decrease the expression of the catalytic subunit of glutamine-cysteine ligase (GCLC) was found in increased levels in the plasma samples from individuals with T2DM, explaining the possible underlying mechanism that is responsible for decreased levels of GSH in individuals with T2DM. Moreover, increased levels of pro-inflammatory cytokines such as interleukin-6 (IL-6) and interleukin-17 (IL-17) were observed in plasma samples isolated from individuals with T2DM. Increased levels of IL-6 and IL-17 was accompanied by enhanced production of free radicals further indicating an alternative mechanism for the decreased levels of GSH in individuals with T2DM. **Augmenting the levels of GSH in macrophages isolated from individuals with T2DM resulted in improved control of M. tb infection. Furthermore, cytokines that are responsible for controlling M. tb infection at the cellular and granuloma level such as tumor necrosis factor alpha (TNF-α), interleukin-1β (IL-1β), interleukin-2 (IL-2), interferon-gamma (IFN-γ), and interleukin-12 (IL-12), were found to be compromised in plasma samples isolated from individuals with T2DM.** On the other hand, interleukin-10 (IL-10), an immunosuppressive cytokine was increased in plasma samples isolated from individuals with T2DM. **Overall, these findings suggest that lower levels of GSH in individuals with T2DM lead to their increased susceptibility to M. tb infection.**

PMID: 25790445 PMCID: PMC4366217 DOI: 10.1371/journal.pone.0118436

Fiziol Zh. **2013;59(2):92-5.**

[Changes in the content of reduced glutathione in severe injuries and multiple trauma].

[Article in Ukrainian]

Pidruchna SR.

Abstract

We explored the changes in reduced glutathione in pathogenesis of severe and combined trauma. Under conditions of our experiments both in blood plasma and tissue of liver, kidneys and heart the concentration of reduced glutathione is decreased. Comparison of the changes ofglutathione that occur in animals of the first experimental group (only severe group) with the same in animals of the second and the third groups, caused by the influence of extra mechanical defect and skin burn, showed that in the last group the disorders of functional status system of antioxidant protection occur more often than in only severely injured animals. **The largest significant decrease (34%) in the content of GSH on the 3rd day after injury we found in liver of seriously injured burned animals.** In animals of the first and second groups the content of GSH decreased by 27 and 33.7%, respectively.

Eur J Trauma Emerg Surg. 2016 Dec;42(6):775-783. Epub 2015 Nov 27.

Efficacy of glutathione mesotherapy in burns: an experimental study.

Buz A[1], Görgülü T[2], Olgun A[1], Kargi E[1].

Author information

Abstract
BACKGROUND:
Thermal burns are the leading cause of trauma worldwide. Currently, no consensus on optimal treatment of deep partial-thickness (second-degree) burns has emerged, as reflected by the wide variability in available wound-care materials. The relative efficacies of products used for treatment of partial-thickness thermal burns remain unclear. Mesotherapy features intradermal administration of various agents, depending on burn location. In the present experimental study, we explored the efficacy of mesotherapy used to treat partial-thickness thermal burns in 50 male Wistar rats divided into five groups of equal number. No procedure was performed after infliction of thermal burns in control group (Group 1). Mesotherapy was applied with physiological saline in sham group (Group 2), glutathione, taurine, and L-carnitine were separately applied in Group 3, Group 4, and Group 5, respectively.

MATERIALS AND METHODS:

Mesotherapeutic agents were injected intradermally into the reticular layer of the dermis using the point technique. The first course of mesotherapy was given within the first 2 h after infliction of thermal burns, and therapy was continued to day 10. On day 22, unhealed thermal burn areas were measured prior to sacrifice, and biopsies covering the total areas of burns were performed to allow of pathological evaluation.

RESULTS:

Group 3 (the glutathione group) showed the best extent of healing, followed by Group 4 (the taurine group) and Group 5 (the L-carnitine group). The healed thermal burn areas in these groups were significantly greater than those in the control and sham groups $(P = 0.001)$. All of healing, acute and chronic inflammation, the amount of granulation tissue, the level of fibroblast maturation, the amount of collagen, the extent of re-epithelization and neovascularization, and ulcer depth were scored upon pathological examination of tissue cross-sections. The best outcomes were evident in the glutathione group, with statistical significance. Although wound healing in the L-carnitine and taurine groups was better than in the control and sham groups, the differences were not statistically significant.

CONCLUSION:

Thus, glutathione mesotherapy was effective when used to treat partial-thickness thermal burns and may be a useful treatment option for various human burns.

EMBO Mol Med. 2016 Nov 17. pii: e201606356. doi: 10.15252/emmm.201606356. [Epub ahead of print]

Coenzyme Q deficiency causes impairment of the sulfide oxidation pathway.

Ziosi M1, Di Meo I2, Kleiner G1, Gao XH3, Barca E1,4, Sanchez-Quintero MJ1, Tadesse S1, Jiang H5, Qiao C5, Rodenburg RJ6, Scalais E7, Schuelke M8, Willard B9, Hatzoglou M3, Tiranti V10, Quinzii CM11.

Author information

Abstract

Coenzyme Q (CoQ) is an electron acceptor for sulfide-quinone reductase (SQR), the first enzyme of the hydrogen sulfide oxidation pathway. Here, we show that lack of CoQ in human skin fibroblasts causes impairment of hydrogen sulfide oxidation, proportional to the residual levels of CoQ. Biochemical and molecular abnormalities are rescued by CoQ supplementation in vitro and recapitulated by pharmacological inhibition of CoQ biosynthesis in skin fibroblasts and ADCK3 depletion in HeLa cells. Kidneys of Pdss2kd/kd mice, which only have ~15% residual CoQ concentrations and are clinically affected, showed (i) reduced protein levels of SQR and downstream enzymes, (ii) accumulation of hydrogen sulfides, and (iii) glutathione depletion. These abnormalities were not present in brain, which maintains ~30% residual CoQ and is clinically unaffected. In Pdss2kd/kd mice, we also observed low levels of plasma and urine thiosulfate and increased blood C4-C6 acylcarnitines. **We propose that impairment of the sulfide oxidation pathway induced by decreased levels of CoQ causes accumulation of sulfides and consequent inhibition of short-chain acyl-CoA dehydrogenase and glutathione depletion, which contributes to increased oxidative stress and kidney failure.**

KEYWORDS:

SQR ; CoQ10; Pdss2; coenzyme Q; sulfides

PMID: 27856618 DOI: 10.15252/emmm.201606356

Blood. 2007 Apr 15;109(8):3560-6. Epub 2006 Dec 21.

Molecular basis of glutathione reductase deficiency in human blood cells.

Kamerbeek NM1, van Zwieten R, de Boer M, Morren G, Vuil H, Bannink N, Lincke C, Dolman KM, Becker K, Schirmer RH, Gromer S, Roos D.

Author information

Abstract

Hereditary glutathione reductase (GR) deficiency was found in only 2 cases when testing more than 15 000 blood samples. We have investigated the blood cells of 2 patients (1a and 1b) in a previously described family suffering from favism and cataract and of a novel patient (2) presenting with severe neonatal jaundice. Red blood cells and leukocytes of the patients in family 1 did not contain any GR activity, and the GR protein was undetectable by Western blotting. Owing to a 2246-bp deletion in the patients' DNA, translated GR is expected to lack almost the complete dimerization domain, which results in unstable and inactive enzyme. The red blood cells from patient 2 did not exhibit GR activity either, but the patient's leukocytes contained some residual activity that correlated with a weak protein expression. Patient 2 was found to be a compound heterozygote, with a premature stop codon on one allele and a substitution of glycine 330, a highly conserved residue in the superfamily of NAD(P)H-dependent disulfide reductases, into alanine on the other allele. Studies on recombinant GR G330A revealed a drastically impaired thermostability of the protein. This is the first identification of mutations in the GR gene causing clinical GR deficiency.

PMID: 17185460 DOI: 10.1182/blood-2006-08-042531

GSTP1provided by HGNC

Official Full Name

glutathione S-transferase pi 1provided by HGNC

Primary source

HGNC:HGNC:4638

See related

Ensembl:ENSG00000084207 HPRD:00614; MIM:134660; Vega:OTTHUMG00000137430

Gene type

protein coding

RefSeq status

REVIEWED

Organism

Homo sapiens

Lineage

Eukaryota; Metazoa; Chordata; Craniata; Vertebrata; Euteleostomi; Mammalia; Eutheria; Euarchontoglires; Primates; Haplorrhini; Catarrhini; Hominidae; Homo

Also known as

PI; DFN7; GST3; GSTP; FAEES3; HEL-S-22

Summary

Glutathione S-transferases (GSTs) are a family of enzymes that play an important role in detoxification by catalyzing the conjugation of many hydrophobic and electrophilic compounds with reduced glutathione. Based on their biochemical, immunologic, and structural properties, the soluble GSTs are categorized into 4 main classes: alpha, mu, pi, and theta. This GST family member is a polymorphic gene encoding active, functionally different GSTP1 variant proteins that are thought to function in xenobiotic metabolism and play a role in susceptibility to cancer, and other diseases. [provided by RefSeq, Jul 2008]

GPX1provided by HGNC

Official Full Name

glutathione peroxidase 1provided by HGNC

Primary source

HGNC:HGNC:4553

See related

Ensembl:ENSG00000233276 HPRD:11749; MIM:138320; Vega:OTTHUMG00000156837

Gene type

protein coding

RefSeq status

REVIEWED

Organism

Homo sapiens

Lineage

Eukaryota; Metazoa; Chordata; Craniata; Vertebrata; Euteleostomi; Mammalia; Eutheria; Euarchontoglires; Primates; Haplorrhini; Catarrhini; Hominidae; Homo

Also known as

GPXD; GSHPX1

Summary

The protein encoded by this gene belongs to the glutathione peroxidase family, members of which catalyze the reduction of organic hydroperoxides and hydrogen peroxide ($H2O2$) by glutathione, and thereby protect cells against oxidative damage. Other studies indicate that $H2O2$ is also essential for growth-factor mediated signal transduction, mitochondrial function, and maintenance of thiol redox-balance; therefore, by limiting $H2O2$ accumulation, glutathione peroxidases are also involved in modulating these processes. Several isozymes of this gene family exist in vertebrates, which vary in cellular location and substrate specificity. This isozyme is the most abundant, is ubiquitously expressed and localized in the cytoplasm, and whose preferred substrate is hydrogen peroxide. It is also a selenoprotein, containing the rare amino acid selenocysteine (Sec) at its active site. Sec is encoded by the UGA codon, which normally signals translation termination. The 3' UTRs of selenoprotein mRNAs contain a conserved stem-loop structure, designated the Sec insertion sequence (SECIS) element, that is necessary for the recognition of UGA as a Sec codon, rather than as a stop signal. This gene contains an in-frame GCG trinucleotide repeat in the coding region, and three alleles with 4, 5 or 6 repeats have been found in the human population. The allele with 4 GCG repeats has been significantly associated with breast cancer risk in premenopausal women. Alternatively spliced transcript variants and multiple pseudogenes of this gene have been identified. [provided by RefSeq, Jul 2016]

J Altern Complement Med. 2011 Sep;17(9):827-33. doi: 10.1089/acm.2010.0716.

Effects of oral glutathione supplementation on systemic oxidative stress biomarkers in human volunteers.

Allen J, Bradley RD.

Abstract

BACKGROUND:

The tripeptide glutathione (GSH) is the most abundant free radical scavenger synthesized endogenously in humans. Increasing mechanistic, clinical, and epidemiological evidence demonstrates that GSH status is significant in acute and chronic diseases. Despite ease of delivery, little controlled clinical research data exist evaluating the effects of oral GSH supplementation.

OBJECTIVES:

The study objectives were to determine the effect of oral GSH supplementation on biomarkers of systemic oxidative stress in human volunteers.

DESIGN:

This was a randomized, double-blind, placebo-controlled clinical trial.

SETTING/LOCATION:

The study was conducted at Bastyr University

Research Institute, Kenmore, WA and the Bastyr Center for Natural Health, Seattle, WA.

SUBJECTS:

Forty(40) adult volunteers without acute or chronic disease participated in this study.

INTERVENTION:

Oral GSH supplementation (500 mg twice daily) was given to the volunteers for 4 weeks.

OUTCOME MEASURES: Primary outcome measures included change in creatinine-standardized, urinary F2-isoprostanes (F2-isoP) and urinary 8-hydroxy-2'-deoxyguanosine (8-OHdG). Changes in erythrocyte GSH concentrations, including total reduced glutathione (GSH), oxidized glutathione (GSSG), and their ratio (GSH:GSSG) were also measured by tandem liquid chromatography/mass spectrometry. Analysis of variance was used to evaluate differences between groups.

RESULTS: There were no differences in oxidative stress biomarkers between treatment groups at baseline. Thirty-nine (39) participants completed the study per protocol. Changes in creatinine standardized F2-isoP (ng/mg creatinine) (0.0 ± 0.1 versus 0.0 ± 0.1, p=0.38) and 8-OHdG (μg/g creatinine) (-0.2 ± 3.3 versus 1.0 ± 3.2, p=0.27) were nonsignificant between groups at week 4. Total reduced, oxidized, and ratio measures of GSH status were also unchanged.

CONCLUSIONS:

No significant changes were observed in biomarkers of oxidative stress, including glutathione status, in this clinical trial of oral glutathione supplementation in healthy adults.

PMID: 21875351 PMCID: PMC3162377 DOI: 10.1089/acm.2010.0716

Biol Trace Elem Res. 2016 Mar;170(1):1-8. doi: 10.1007/s12011-015-0435-z. Epub 2015 Jul 17.

The Level of Selenium and Oxidative Stress in Workers Chronically Exposed to Lead.

Pawlas N1, Dobrakowski M2, Kasperczyk A2, Kozłowska A1, Mikołajczyk A1, Kasperczyk S3.

Author information

Abstract

The possible beneficial role of selenium (Se) on the oxidative stress induced by lead (Pb) is still unclear in humans. Therefore, the aim of the present study was to explore the associations among the Se levels, chronic Pb exposure, oxidative stress parameters, and parameters characterizing the function of the antioxidant defense system in men who are occupationally exposed to Pb. Based on the median serum Se concentrations, the 324 study subjects were divided into two subgroups: a subgroup with a low Se level (L-Se) and a subgroup with a high Se level (H-Se). The levels of lead (PbB) and zinc protoporphyrin (ZPP) in the blood and the delta-aminolevulinic acid (ALA) level in the urine served as indices of Pb exposure. The PbB level was significantly lower in the H-Se group compared to that in the L-Se group by 6 %. The levels of 8-hydroxyguanosine and lipofuscin (LPS) and the activity of superoxide dismutase were significantly lower in the H-Se group compared to that in the L-Se group by 17, 19, and 11 %, respectively. However, the glutathione level (GSH) and the activities of glutathione peroxidase (GPx) and catalase were significantly higher by 9, 23, and 3 %. Spearman correlations showed positive associations between the Se level and GPx activity and GSH level. A lower serum Se level in chronically Pb-exposed subjects is associated with higher Pb blood levels and an elevated erythrocyte LPS level, which reflects the intensity of oxidative stress. Besides, in a group of Pb-exposed subjects with lower serum Se level, depleted GSH pool and decreased activity of GPx in erythrocytes were reported. However, the present results are inadequate to recommend Se supplementation for chronic lead exposure at higher doses than would be included in a normal diet except for selenium deficiency.

KEYWORDS:

Antioxidant defense system; Glutathione peroxidase; Lead poisoning; Oxidative stress; Selenium

PMID: 26179085 PMCID: PMC4744245 DOI: 10.1007/s12011-015-0435-z

Free Radic Biol Med. 2013 Dec;65:488-96. doi: 10.1016/j.freeradbiomed.2013.07.021. Epub 2013 Jul 26.

Impaired synthesis and antioxidant defense of glutathione in the cerebellum of autistic subjects: alterations in the activities and protein expression of glutathione-related enzymes.

Gu F1, Chauhan V, Chauhan A.

Author information

Abstract

Autism is a neurodevelopmental disorder associated with social deficits and behavioral abnormalities. Recent evidence in autism suggests a deficit in glutathione (GSH), a major endogenous antioxidant. It is not known whether the synthesis, consumption, and/or regeneration of GSH is affected in autism. In the cerebellum tissues from autism (n=10) and age-matched control subjects (n=10), the activities of GSH-related enzymes glutathione peroxidase (GPx), glutathione-S-transferase (GST), glutathione reductase (GR), and glutamate cysteine ligase (GCL) involved in antioxidant defense, detoxification, GSH regeneration, and synthesis, respectively, were analyzed. GCL is a rate-limiting enzyme for GSH synthesis, and the relationship between its activity and the protein expression of its catalytic subunit GCLC and its modulatory subunit GCLM was also compared between the autistic and the control groups. Results showed that the activities of GPx and GST were significantly decreased in autism compared to that of the control group (P<0.05). Although there was no significant difference in GR activity between autism and control groups, 40% of autistic subjects showed lower GR activity than 95% confidence interval (CI) of the control group. GCL activity was also significantly reduced by 38.7% in the autistic group compared to the control group (P=0.023), and 8 of 10 autistic subjects had values below 95% CI of the control group. The ratio of protein levels of GCLC to GCLM in the autism group was significantly higher than that of the control group (P=0.022), and GCLM protein levels were reduced by 37.3% in the autistic group compared to the control group. A positive strong correlation was observed between GCL activity and protein levels of GCLM (r=0.887) and GCLC (r=0.799) subunits in control subjects but not in autistic subjects, suggesting that regulation of GCL activity is affected in autism. These results suggest that enzymes involved in GSH homeostasis have impaired activities in the cerebellum in autism, and lower GCL activity in autism may be related to decreased protein expression of GCLM.

KEYWORDS:

2,3-naphthalenedicarboxyaldehyde; ASDs; Autism; Brain; Cerebellum; GCL; GPx; GR; GST; Glutamate cysteine ligase; Glutathione; Glutathione S-transferase; Glutathione peroxidase; Glutathione reductase; NDA; Oxidative stress; PKA; PKC; ROS; autism spectrum disorders; glutamate cysteine ligase; glutathione peroxidase; glutathione reductase; glutathione-S-transferase; protein kinase A; protein kinase C; reactive oxygen species.

PMID: 23892356 DOI: 10.1016/j.freeradbiomed.2013.07.021

Mol Autism. 2016 Apr 21;7:26. doi: 10.1186/s13229-016-0088-6. eCollection 2016.

A randomized placebo-controlled pilot study of N-acetylcysteine in youth with autism spectrum disorder.

Wink LK1, Adams R1, Wang Z2, Klaunig JE2, Plawecki MH3, Posey DJ4, McDougle CJ5, Erickson CA1.

Author information

Abstract

BACKGROUND:

Social impairment is a defining feature of autism spectrum disorder (ASD) with no demonstrated effective pharmacologic treatments. The goal of this study was to evaluate efficacy, safety, and tolerability of oral N-acetylcysteine (NAC), an antioxidant whose function overlaps with proposed mechanisms of ASD pathophysiology, targeting core social impairment in youth with ASD.

METHODS:

This study was a 12-week randomized, double-blind, placebo-controlled trial of oral NAC in youth with ASD. Study participants were medically healthy youth age 4 to 12 years with ASD, weighing ≥15 kg, and judged to be moderately ill based on the Clinical Global Impressions Severity scale. The participants were randomized via computer to active drug or placebo in a 1:1 ratio, with the target dose of NAC being 60 mg/kg/day in three divided doses. The primary outcome measure of efficacy was the Clinical Global Impressions Improvement (CGI-I) scale anchored to core social impairment. To investigate the impact of NAC on oxidative stress markers in peripheral blood, venous blood samples were collected at screen and week 12.

RESULTS:

Thirty-one patients were enrolled (NAC = 16, placebo = 15). Three participants were lost to follow-up, and three left the trial due to adverse effects. The average daily dose of NAC at week 12 was 56.2 mg/kg (SD = 9.7) with dose ranging from 33.6 to 64.3 mg/kg. The frequency of adverse events was so low that comparisons between groups could not be conducted. At week 12, there was no statistically significant difference between the NAC and placebo groups on the CGI-I ($p > 0.69$) but the glutathione (GSH) level in blood was significantly higher in the NAC group ($p < 0.05$). The oxidative glutathione disulfide (GSSG) level increased in the NAC group, however only at a trend level of significance ($p = 0.09$). There was no significant difference between the NAC and placebo groups in the GSH/GSSG ratio, DNA strand break and oxidative damage, and blood homocysteine levels at week 12 (ps > 0.16).

CONCLUSIONS:

The results of this trial indicate that NAC treatment was well tolerated, had the expected effect of boosting GSH production, but had no significant impact on social impairment in youth with ASD.

TRIAL REGISTRATION:

Clinicaltrials.gov NCT00453180.

KEYWORDS:

Autism; Autism spectrum disorder; N-acetylcysteine; Oxidative stress; Social impairment

PMID: 27103982 PMCID: PMC4839099 DOI: 10.1186/s13229-016-0088-6

Dig Dis. 2015;33(4):464-71. doi: 10.1159/000374090. Epub 2015 Jul 6.

Acetaminophen: Dose-Dependent Drug Hepatotoxicity and Acute Liver Failure in Patients.

Jaeschke H1.

Author information

Abstract

BACKGROUND:

Drug-induced liver injury is a rare but serious clinical problem. A number of drugs can cause severe liver injury and acute liver failure at therapeutic doses in a very limited number of patients (<1:10,000). This idiosyncratic drug-induced liver injury, which is currently not predictable in preclinical safety studies, appears to depend on individual susceptibility and the inability to adapt to the cellular stress caused by a particular drug. In striking contrast to idiosyncratic drug-induced liver injury, drugs with dose-dependent hepatotoxicity are mostly detected during preclinical studies and do not reach the market. One notable exception is acetaminophen (APAP, paracetamol), which is a safe drug at therapeutic doses but can cause severe liver injury and acute liver failure after intentional and unintentional overdoses. Key Messages: APAP overdose is responsible for more acute liver failure cases in the USA or UK than all other etiologies combined. Since APAP overdose in the mouse represents a model for the human pathophysiology, substantial progress has been made during the last decade in understanding the mechanisms of cell death, liver injury and recovery. More recently, emerging evidence based on mechanistic biomarker analysis in patients and studies of cell death in human hepatocytes suggests that most of the mechanisms discovered in mice also apply to patients. The rapid development of N-acetylcysteine as an antidote against APAP overdose was based on the early understanding of APAP toxicity in mice. However, despite the efficacy of N-acetylcysteine in patients who present early after APAP overdose, there is a need to develop intervention strategies for late-presenting patients.

CONCLUSIONS:

The challenges related to APAP toxicity are to better understand the mechanisms of cell death in order to limit liver injury and prevent acute liver failure, and also to develop biomarkers that better predict as early as possible who is at risk for developing acute liver failure with poor outcome.

© 2015 S. Karger AG, Basel.

PMID: 26159260 PMCID: PMC4520394 DOI: 10.1159/000374090

Neurochem Int. 2000 Apr;36(4-5):461-9.

The glutathione content of retinal Müller (glial) cells: effect of pathological conditions.

Huster D1, Reichenbach A, Reichelt W.

Author information

Abstract

Maintenance of isolated retinal Müller (glial) cells in glutamate-free solutions over 7 h causes a significant loss of their initial glutathione content; this loss is largely prevented by the blockade of glutamine synthesis using methionine sulfoximine (5 mM). Anoxia does not reduce the glutathione content of Müller cells when glucose (11 mM), glutamate and cystine (0.1 mM each) are present. In contrast, simulation of total ischemia (i.e., anoxia plus removal of glucose) decreases the glutathione levels dramatically, even in the presence of glutamate and cystine. Less severe effects are caused by high extracellular K+ (40 mM). Reactive oxygen species are generated in the retina under various conditions, such as anoxia, ischemia, and reperfusion. One of the crucial substances protecting the retina against reactive oxygen species is glutathione, a tripeptide constituted of glutamate, cysteine and glycine. It was recently shown that glutathione can be synthesized in retinal Müller glial cells and that glutamate is the rate-limiting substance. In this study, glutathione levels were determined in acutely isolated guinea-pig Müller cells using the glutathione-sensitive fluorescent dye monochlorobimane. The purpose was to find out how the glial glutathione content is affected by anoxia/ischemia and accompanying pathophysiological events such as depolarization of the cell membrane. **Our results further strengthen the view that glutamate is rate-limiting for the glutathione synthesis in glial cells.** During glutamate deficiency, as caused by e.g., impaired glutamate uptake, this amino acid is preferentially delivered to the glutamate-glutamine pathway, at the expense of glutathione. This mechanism may contribute to the finding that total ischemia (but not anoxia) causes a depletion of glial glutathione. In situ depletion may be accelerated by the ischemia-induced increase of extracellular K+, decreasing the driving force for glutamate uptake. The ischemia-induced lack of glutathione is particularly fatal considering the increased production of reactive oxygen species under this condition. Therefore the therapeutic application of exogenous free radical scavengers is greatly recommended.

PMID: 10733014

Biol Chem. 2016 Sep 14. pii: /j/bchm.ahead-of-print/hsz-2016-0202/hsz-2016-0202.xml. doi: 10.1515/hsz-2016-0202. [Epub ahead of print]

Glutathione and glutathione derivatives in immunotherapy.

Fraternale A, Brundu S, Magnani M.

Abstract

Reduced glutathione (GSH) is the most prevalent non-protein thiol in animal cells. Its de novo and salvage synthesis serves to maintain a reduced cellular environment, which is important for several cellular functions. Altered intracellular GSH levels are observed in a wide range of pathologies, including several viral infections, as well as in aging, all of which are also characterized by an unbalanced Th1/Th2 immune response. **A central role in influencing the immune response has been ascribed to GSH.** Specifically, GSH depletion in antigen-presenting cells (APCs) correlates with altered antigen processing and reduced secretion of Th1 cytokines. Conversely, an increase in intracellular GSH content stimulates IL-12 and/or IL-27, which in turn induces differentiation of naive CD4+ T cells to Th1 cells. In addition, **GSH has been shown to inhibit the replication/survival of several pathogens, i.e. viruses and bacteria.** Hence, molecules able to increase GSH levels have been proposed as new tools to more effectively hinder different pathogens by acting as both immunomodulators and antimicrobials. Herein, the new role of GSH and its derivatives as immunotherapeutics will be discussed.

PMID: 27514076 DOI: 10.1515/hsz-2016-0202

J Strength Cond Res. 2016 Jul 25. [Epub ahead of print]

Variations In Oxidative Stress Levels In Three Days Follow-Up In Ultra-Marathon Mountain Race Athletes.

Ypatios S1, Dimitrios S, Marina O, Nikolaos G, David BO, Demetrios S, Demetrios K.

Author information

Abstract

The aim of the present study was the monitoring of the redox status of runners participating in a mountain ultra-marathon race of 103 km. Blood samples from 12 runners were collected pre race and 24, 48 and 72 h post race. The samples were analyzed by using conventional oxidative stress markers, such as protein carbonyls (CARB), thiobarbituric acid reactive substances (TBARS), total antioxidant capacity (TAC) in plasma, as well as glutathione (GSH) levels and catalase (CAT) activity in erythrocytes. In addition, two novel markers the static oxidation-reduction potential marker (sORP) and the capacity oxidation-reduction potential (cORP) were measured in plasma. The results showed significant increase in sORP levels and significant decrease in cORP and GSH levels post race compared to pre race. The other markers did not exhibit significant changes post race compared to pre race. Furthermore, an inter-individual analysis showed that in all athletes but one sORP was increased, while cORP was decreased. Moreover, GSH levels were decreased in all athletes at least at two time points post race compared to pre race. The other markers exhibited great variations between different athletes. In conclusion, ORP and GSH markers suggested that oxidative stress has existed even 3 days post ultra-marathon race. The practical applications from these results would be that the most effective markers for short-term monitoring of ultra-marathon mountain race-induced oxidative stress were sORP, cORP and GSH. Also, administration of supplements enhancing especially GSH is recommended during ultra-marathon mountain races in order to prevent manifestation of pathological conditions.

PMID: 27465629 DOI: 10.1519/JSC.0000000000001584

Chapter 12

Final Thoughts on VARS

We did it.

As I write this we have a patent pending on the first Liposoal Reduced Stable Glutathione.

It is named VARS® Liposomal Glutathione – VARS stands for Validated, Absorbable, Reduced and Stable. VARS® increases GSH levels 41% on the first day of use with only ONE application/dose – that is insane. There's nothing like it on the planet.

I hope and pray that it will save a lot of lives and improve the quality of life all over the planet.

Thanks for reading.

– Dan Purser MD

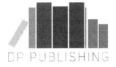

PhysicianDesigned.com

DanPurserMD.com

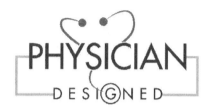

[1] No author listed. Accessed on line 7 Dec 2016 at http://www.fda.gov/Cosmetics/GuidanceRegulation/LawsRegulations/ucm074201.htm

[2] Allen J, Bradley RD. Effects of oral glutathione supplementation on systemic oxidative stress biomarkers in human volunteers. J Altern Complement Med. 2011 Sep;17(9):827-33. doi: 10.1089/acm.2010.0716.

[3] No author listed. Accessed 18 Dec 2016 online at http://www.essentialgsh.com/Glutathione.html

[4] SNOKE JE, YANARI S, BLOCH K. Synthesis of glutathione from gamma-glutamylcysteine. J Biol Chem. 1953 Apr;201(2):573-86.

[5] Gu F, Chauhan V, Chauhan A. Impaired synthesis and antioxidant defense of glutathione in the cerebellum of autistic subjects: alterations in the activities and protein expression of glutathione-related enzymes. Free Radic Biol Med. 2013 Dec;65:488-96. doi: 10.1016/j.freeradbiomed.2013.07.021.

[6] Peck, M. Epidemiology of burn injuries globally. Accessed 18 Dec 2016 at http://www.uptodate.com/contents/epidemiology-of-burn-injuries-globally

[7] Buz A, Görgülü T, Olgun A, Kargi E. Efficacy of glutathione mesotherapy in burns: an experimental study. Eur J Trauma Emerg Surg. 2016 Dec;42(6):775-783.

[8] Lozano-Sepulveda SA, Bryan-Marrugo OL, et al. Oxidative stress modulation in hepatitis C virus infected cells. World J Hepatol. 2015 Dec 18;7(29):2880-9. doi: 10.4254/wjh.v7.i29.2880.

[9] Stephensen CB, Marquis GS, et al. Glutathione, glutathione peroxidase, and selenium status in HIV-positive and HIV-negative adolescents and young adults. Am J Clin Nutr. 2007 Jan;85(1):173-81.

[10] Krezel A1, Bal W. Studies of zinc(II) and nickel(II) complexes of GSH, GSSG and their analogs shed more light on their biological relevance. Bioinorg Chem Appl. 2004:293-305. doi:

10.1155/S1565363304000172.

[11] Paşca SP, Nemeş B, et al. High levels of homocysteine and low serum paraoxonase 1 arylesterase activity in children with autism. Life Sci. 2006 Apr 4;78(19):2244-8.

[12] Kumawat M1, Sharma TK, et al. N Am J Med Sci. 2013 Mar;5(3):213-9. doi: 10.4103/1947-2714.109193. Antioxidant Enzymes and Lipid Peroxidation in Type 2 Diabetes Mellitus Patients with and without Nephropathy.

[13] Allen J, Bradley RD. Effects of oral glutathione supplementation on systemic oxidative stress biomarkers in human volunteers. J Altern Complement Med. 2011 Sep;17(9):827-33. doi: 10.1089/acm.2010.0716.

[14] Alfthan G. Xu GL. Tan WH. Aro A. Wu J. Yang YX. Liang WS. Xue WL. Kong LH. Selenium supplementation of children in a selenium-deficient area in China: blood selenium levels and glutathione peroxidase activities. Biol Trace Elem Res. 2000;73:113–125.

[15] Fuyu Y. Keshan disease and mitochondrial cardiomyopathy. Sci China C Life Sci. 2006;49:513–518.

[16] Lei C. Niu X. Wei J. Zhu J. Zhu Y. Interaction of glutathione peroxidase-1 and selenium in endemic dilated cardiomyopathy. Clin Chim Acta. 2009;399:102–108.

[17] Reeves WC. Marcuard SP. Willis SE. Movahed A. Reversible cardiomyopathy due to selenium deficiency. JPEN J Parenter Enteral Nutr. 1989;13:663–665.

[18] Peng A. Yang C. Rui H. Li H. Study on the pathogenic factors of Kashin-Beck disease. J Toxicol Environ Health. 1992;35:79–90.

[19] Wu J. Xu GL. Plasma selenium content, platelet glutathione peroxidase and superoxide dismutase activity of residents in Kashin-Beck disease affected area in China. J Trace Elem Electrolytes Health Dis. 1987;1:39–43

[20] Lubos E, Kelly NJ, et al. J Biol Chem. 2011 Oct 14;286(41):35407-17. doi: 10.1074/jbc.M110.205708. Glutathione peroxidase-1 deficiency augments proinflammatory

cytokine-induced redox signaling and human endothelial cell activation.

[21] Islam MT. Oxidative stress and mitochondrial dysfunction-linked neurodegenerative disorders. Neurol Res. 2017 Jan;39(1):73-82.

[22] Bailey BO. Acetaminophen hepatotoxicity and overdose. Am Fam Physician. 1980 Jul;22(1):83-7.

[23] Whitehouse LW, Wong LT, et al. Postabsorption antidotal effects of N-acetylcysteine on acetaminophen-induced hepatotoxicity in the mouse. Can J Physiol Pharmacol. 1985 May;63(5):431-7.

[24] Lőrincz T1, Jemnitz K, et al. Ferroptosis is Involved in Acetaminophen Induced Cell Death. Pathol Oncol Res. 2015 Sep;21(4):1115-21. doi: 10.1007/s12253-015-9946-3.

[25] No author listed. Accessed 17 Dec 2016 online at https://www.healthaliciousness.com/articles/high-cysteine-foods.php.

[26] Axe, J. 9 Ways to Boost Glutathione. Accessed 17 Dec 2016 online at https://draxe.com/glutathione/.

[27] No author listed. Accessed 17 Dec 2016 online at healthyeating.sfgate.com/food-sources-alphalipoic-acid-1552.html.

[28] Kerasioti E, Stagos D, et al. Antioxidant Effects of Sheep Whey Protein on Endothelial Cells. Oxid Med Cell Longev. 2016;2016:6585737. doi: 10.1155/2016/6585737.

[29] Li C, Zhang WJ, et al. Quercetin affects glutathione levels and redox ratio in human aortic endothelial cells not through oxidation but formation and cellular export of quercetin-glutathione conjugates and upregulation of glutamate-cysteine ligase. Redox Biol. 2016 Oct;9:220-228. doi: 10.1016/j.redox.2016.08.012.

Made in the USA
Las Vegas, NV
02 February 2021